DEALING
WITH
TYPE 2
DIABETES

A Holistic Guide to Navigating the Journey with Low Carb, Low Sugar Solutions, Balanced Nutrition, and Empowering Lifestyle Strategies

+   Bonus: 30 days meal plan

Dr. Edna Swindell, MD

Copyright

Disclaimer

This book is provided for general informational purposes only and does not constitute medical advice. The author and publisher are not responsible for any consequences resulting from the use of information contained in this book. Readers are advised to consult with a qualified healthcare professional for medical advice, diagnosis, and treatment tailored to their specific needs.

The information in this book is based on the author's professional experience and extensive research at the time of writing. Medical knowledge is constantly evolving, and new developments may arise. The author and publisher disclaim any responsibility for errors or omissions or for any consequences arising from the use of the information contained herein.

Every effort has been made to ensure the accuracy of the information presented. However, the author and publisher do not guarantee the accuracy, completeness, or usefulness of the information and are not responsible for any errors or omissions.

HERE IS YOUR BONUS

30-Day Meal Plan to get you started!. All recipes and processes for preparing are discussed later in this book

Week 1:

Day 1:

- Breakfast: Scrambled eggs with spinach and tomatoes
- Lunch: Grilled chicken salad with mixed greens, cherry tomatoes, and vinaigrette
- Dinner: Baked salmon with lemon and herbs, steamed broccoli

Day 2:

- Breakfast: Greek yogurt with berries and a sprinkle of nuts
- Lunch: Turkey and avocado lettuce wraps
- Dinner: Cauliflower rice stir-fry with tofu and mixed vegetables

Day 3:

- Breakfast: Chia seed pudding with almond milk and sliced strawberries
- Lunch: Quinoa salad with chickpeas, cucumbers, and feta cheese
- Dinner: Grilled shrimp skewers with asparagus

Day 4:

- Breakfast: Omelette with mushrooms, bell peppers, and cheese
- Lunch: Spinach and feta stuffed chicken breast, side of roasted Brussels sprouts
- Dinner: Zucchini noodles with tomato and basil sauce, grilled chicken

Day 5:

- Breakfast: Cottage cheese and pineapple bowl
- Lunch: Tuna salad lettuce wraps
- Dinner: Baked cod with a side of sautéed spinach and garlic

Day 6:

- Breakfast: Smoothie with unsweetened almond milk, kale, banana, and protein powder
- Lunch: Egg salad in whole-grain wraps
- Dinner: Turkey meatballs with zucchini noodles

Day 7:

- Breakfast: Avocado and smoked salmon on whole-grain toast
- Lunch: Lentil soup with a side of mixed greens
- Dinner: Grilled chicken breast with roasted sweet potatoes

Week 2:

Day 8:

- Breakfast: Almond flour pancakes with berries
- Lunch: Caprese salad with grilled chicken
- Dinner: Stir-fried tofu with broccoli and snap peas

Day 9:

- Breakfast: Overnight oats with almond milk, nuts, and sliced apple
- Lunch: Shrimp and vegetable skewers with quinoa
- Dinner: Baked tilapia with a side of sautéed kale

Day 10:

- Breakfast: Whole-grain toast with mashed avocado and poached eggs
- Lunch: Chicken Caesar salad with a light dressing
- Dinner: Spaghetti squash with turkey bolognese

Day 11:

- Breakfast: Berry and spinach smoothie with protein powder
- Lunch: Chickpea and vegetable curry
- Dinner: Grilled swordfish with a side of roasted Brussels sprouts

Day 12:

- Breakfast: Cottage cheese and sliced peaches

- Breakfast: Cottage cheese and sliced peaches
- Lunch: Turkey and vegetable stir-fry with brown rice
- Dinner: Baked chicken thighs with lemon and herbs, steamed asparagus

Day 13:

- Breakfast: Scrambled tofu with cherry tomatoes and spinach
- Lunch: Avocado and black bean salad
- Dinner: Cod fish tacos with cabbage slaw

Day 14:

- Breakfast: Whole-grain waffles with fresh berries
- Lunch: Egg and vegetable frittata
- Dinner: Grilled lamb chops with a side of roasted sweet potatoes

Week 3:

Day 15:

- Breakfast: Greek yogurt parfait with granola and mixed berries
- Lunch: Spinach and mushroom omelet
- Dinner: Baked chicken with rosemary, quinoa, and steamed broccoli

Day 16:

- Breakfast: Smoothie bowl with kiwi, pineapple, and chia seeds
- Lunch: Quinoa and black bean stuffed peppers
- Dinner: Shrimp scampi with zucchini noodles

Day 17:

- Breakfast: Almond butter and banana on whole-grain toast
- Lunch: Grilled vegetable and feta wrap
- Dinner: Lemon herb marinated grilled chicken with roasted Brussels sprouts

Day 18:

- Breakfast: Chia seed and coconut milk pudding with raspberries
- Lunch: Turkey and vegetable kebabs with a side of quinoa
- Dinner: Baked cod with a lemon herb crust, steamed asparagus

Day 19:

- Breakfast: Oatmeal with sliced strawberries and almonds
- Lunch: Chickpea salad with cucumber, cherry tomatoes, and feta
- Dinner: Grilled vegetable and tofu skewers

Day 20:

- Breakfast: Whole-grain bagel with cream cheese and smoked salmon
- Lunch: Mediterranean salad with grilled chicken
- Dinner: Spaghetti squash primavera with shrimp

Day 21:

- Breakfast: Avocado and egg breakfast wrap
- Lunch: Lentil and vegetable soup with a side of mixed greens
- Dinner: Baked chicken thighs with a balsamic glaze, roasted sweet potatoes

Week 4:

Day 22:

- Breakfast: Yogurt and berry smoothie
- Lunch: Turkey and vegetable lettuce cups
- Dinner: Grilled swordfish with a tomato and cucumber salad

Day 23:

- Breakfast: Almond flour waffles with mixed berries
- Lunch: Quinoa and vegetable bowl with a tahini dressing
- Dinner: Cod fish cakes with a side of sautéed spinach

Day 24:

- Breakfast: Scrambled eggs with mushrooms and bell peppers
- Lunch: Greek chicken souvlaki with a side of tabbouleh
- Dinner: Baked salmon with dill and lemon, steamed broccoli

Day 25:

- Breakfast: Whole-grain toast with mashed avocado and poached eggs

- Lunch: Spinach and feta stuffed chicken breast, side of roasted Brussels sprouts
- Dinner: Zucchini noodles with tomato and basil sauce, grilled chicken

Day 26:

- Breakfast: Cottage cheese and pineapple bowl
- Lunch: Tuna salad lettuce wraps
- Dinner: Baked cod with a side of sautéed spinach and garlic

Day 27:

- Breakfast: Smoothie with unsweetened almond milk, kale, banana, and protein powder
- Lunch: Egg salad in whole-grain wraps
- Dinner: Turkey meatballs with zucchini noodles

Day 28:

- Breakfast: Avocado and smoked salmon on whole-grain toast
- Lunch: Lentil soup with a side of mixed greens
- Dinner: Grilled chicken breast with roasted sweet potatoes

Day 29:

- Breakfast: Almond flour pancakes with berries
- Lunch: Caprese salad with grilled chicken
- Dinner: Stir-fried tofu with broccoli and snap peas

Day 30:

- Breakfast: Overnight oats with almond milk, nuts, and sliced apple
- Lunch: Shrimp and vegetable skewers with quinoa
- Dinner: Baked tilapia with a side of sautéed kale

About the Author

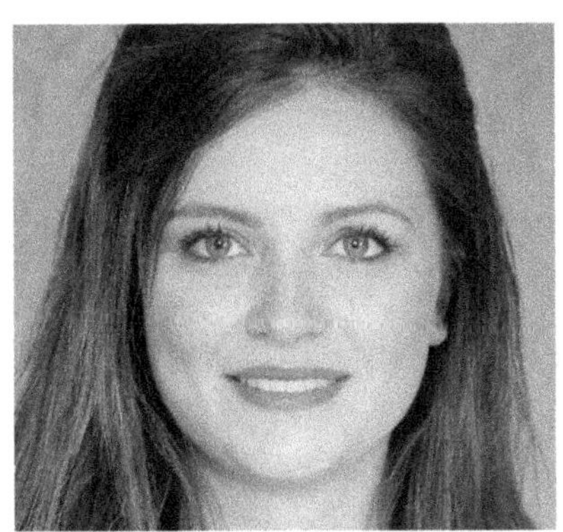

Dr. Edna Swindell, MD

Dr. Edna Swindell is not just an author; she is a seasoned medical professional dedicated to the well-being of individuals and communities. With a passion for health education and a commitment to empowering others with knowledge, Dr. Swindell brings a unique blend of medical expertise and compassionate understanding to the realm of diabetes care.

Medical Journey

As a medical doctor, Dr. Swindell has traversed the corridors of healthcare, accumulating a wealth of experience in patient care, disease management, and health promotion. Her journey has been marked by a genuine concern for the holistic well-being of her patients, leading her to delve into the intricacies of chronic conditions such as Type 2 diabetes.

Passion for Health Education

Driven by a fervor for health education, Dr. Swindell recognized the need for accessible, comprehensible resources to guide individuals on their journeys toward well-being. Through her writing, she seeks to bridge the gap between medical knowledge and everyday understanding, empowering readers to make informed decisions about their health.

Advocate for Empowerment

Dr. Swindell is a strong advocate for empowering individuals in their health journeys. She believes that knowledge is a powerful tool and strives to impart information in a way that is both informative and inspiring. Her commitment to patient education extends beyond the clinic, reaching individuals in the broader community through her written works.

Authorship

Dr. Edna Swindell, channels her medical expertise into authorship, offering readers a compassionate and informed guide in "Dealing with Type 2 Diabetes." This comprehensive work reflects not only her professional knowledge but also her dedication to supporting individuals in managing and thriving with Type 2 diabetes.

Table of Contents

Introduction

Welcome to "Dealing with Type 2 Diabetes: A Holistic Guide to Navigating the Journey with Low Carb, Low Sugar Solutions, Balanced Nutrition, and Empowering Lifestyle Strategies"

In the following pages, we will embark on a journey that will give you the power to take control of your health and manage the difficulties of living with type 2 diabetes with strength and purpose.

Type 2 diabetes is not a sentence; it's an invitation to understand, adapt, and overcome. This guide will be your companion in that journey, providing you with knowledge, strategies, and a 30-day plan that will revolutionize your relationship with diabetes.

Throughout the chapters, this book will explain the complexities of type 2 diabetes, including its causes, the effects of lifestyle choices, and the importance of a balanced diet. At the core of our journey is a carefully designed 30-day meal plan, with low carb and low sugar options that will not only benefit your health but also delight your taste buds.

But this guide is more than just a culinary guide; it's a comprehensive approach to wellness. We will explore the power of physical activity, understand the details of blood sugar monitoring, and address the emotional aspects of living with diabetes. Together, we will create a foundation for long-term well-being.

So, let's take this path with determination, armed with knowledge, and supported by a plan that will not just help you manage but also help you thrive. "Dealing with Type 2 Diabetes" is not just a title; it's a declaration of empowerment. Let's embrace the next 30 days and beyond with resilience, strength, and the belief that you have the power to shape your health.

The journey begins now.

Brief Overview of Type 2 Diabetes

Type 2 diabetes is a metabolic disorder that is characterized by high levels of glucose in the blood. Unlike type 1 diabetes, where the body does not produce insulin, people with type 2 diabetes often produce insulin, but their cells do not respond to it or the pancreas does not make enough. This leads to an imbalance of blood sugar levels, which affects the body's ability to use glucose for energy.

The development of type 2 diabetes is usually caused by a combination of genetic and lifestyle factors. Although there is a hereditary component, environmental factors such as an inactive lifestyle, poor dietary choices, and being overweight can also play a role.

Insulin, a hormone produced by the pancreas, is essential for controlling glucose absorption by cells. In type 2 diabetes, the cells become resistant to insulin, preventing glucose from being taken up efficiently. As a result, glucose accumulates in the bloodstream, leading to hyperglycemia.

Common symptoms of type 2 diabetes include increased thirst, frequent urination, unexplained weight loss, fatigue, and blurred vision. However, some people may not experience any symptoms in the early stages.

Diagnosis is usually confirmed through blood tests, which measure fasting blood sugar levels or glucose tolerance. Once diagnosed, managing type 2 diabetes involves making lifestyle changes, such as eating a balanced diet, exercising regularly, and, in some cases, taking medication.

If left untreated, type 2 diabetes can lead to serious health problems such as heart disease, kidney problems, nerve damage, and vision problems. However, with the right management and a commitment to a healthier lifestyle, people with type 2 diabetes can lead fulfilling lives and reduce the risk of complications. The key to successfully managing type 2 diabetes is to understand its basics and take a holistic approach to wellbeing.

The book encourages readers to celebrate their successes, no matter how small, fostering a positive mindset and reinforcing healthy habits.
Setting sustainable long-term goals is emphasized, ensuring that the changes made over the 30 days are not just short-term adjustments but enduring lifestyle transformations.

10. Empowerment Beyond the Book: Ongoing Resources

The guide doesn't conclude after 30 days; it equips readers with ongoing resources, including a glossary of key terms, additional references, and nutritional information for common foods.
This ensures that readers have the tools they need for continued success beyond the initial 30-day period.

How to Use This book

This book, "Dealing with Type 2 Diabetes: is a great resource to help individuals manage and thrive with type 2 diabetes. To get the most out of it, here are some steps to follow:

1. Start with the Introduction:
Take a look at the introduction to get an understanding of the book's overall philosophy and the journey it encourages you to take.

2. Learn About Type 2 Diabetes:
Start with Chapter 1, "Understanding Type 2 Diabetes," to get the basics of the condition, its causes, and common symptoms.

3. Set Your Goals:
Think about your health goals and intentions for the next 30 days. Use the goal-setting tips in the introduction to set clear and achievable objectives.

4. Follow the 30-Day Action Plan:
Check out Chapter 3 for a detailed overview of the 30-day meal plan. Customize your grocery list based on the sample and explore the low carb, low sugar recipes for breakfast, lunch, dinner, and snacks in Chapter 4.

5. Incorporate Exercise Strategies:
Move on to Chapter 5 to find out the empowering benefits of physical activity. Choose exercise strategies that fit your fitness level and preferences.

6. Monitor Blood Sugar Levels:
Look at Chapter 6 to understand the importance of regular blood sugar monitoring. Learn about blood glucose meters and how to interpret readings accurately.

7. Navigate Medications and Treatment:

Chapter 7 provides insights into medications and treatment options. Understand the role of medications, potential side effects, and the importance of following the treatment plan.

8. Taking Care of Your Emotions:
Head to Chapter 8 for advice on how to manage the emotional struggles that come with type 2 diabetes. Utilize strategies to help you cope with stress and build a strong support system.

9. Avoiding Complications:
Chapter 9 emphasizes the importance of regular check-ups and provides strategies to help you avoid long-term issues.

10. Acknowledging Your Success and Setting Goals:
As you make your way through the 30 days, take the time to recognize your accomplishments. Chapter 10 gives you a framework to reflect, appreciate, and set achievable long-term goals.

11. Utilizing Extra Resources:
Check out the appendices for a list of key terms, extra references, and nutritional information for common foods.

12. Joining the Community:
Think about joining online communities or local support groups to exchange stories, ask questions, and create a network of support.

13. Going Beyond 30 Days:
This guide is the perfect starting point for a lifetime of empowered living. Use the knowledge you gain during the 30 days as a base for continued well-being.

14. Referring Back to the Book:
Keep "Dealing with Type 2 Diabetes" as a reference for ongoing support and motivation. Revisit certain chapters as needed for guidance.

15. Consulting with Healthcare Professionals:

Although this guide is a great resource, always talk to your healthcare team before making major changes to your diet, exercise routine, or medication.

Understanding Type 2 Diabetes: A Comprehensive Exploration

Type 2 diabetes is a prevalent and chronic medical condition that significantly impacts the lives of millions of people worldwide. Characterized by high blood sugar levels, this metabolic disorder arises when the body either resists the effects of insulin or fails to produce enough insulin to maintain normal glucose levels. In this comprehensive exploration, we delve into the intricacies of type 2 diabetes, examining its origins, contributing factors, symptoms, diagnosis, and management strategies.

1. Insulin and Glucose: A Balancing Act

At the heart of type 2 diabetes is the intricate interplay between insulin and glucose. Insulin, a hormone produced by the pancreas, plays a crucial role in regulating the movement of glucose into cells. This process is essential for cells to convert glucose into energy. In individuals with type 2 diabetes, this delicate balance is disrupted.

2. Insulin Resistance and Beta Cell Dysfunction

The development of type 2 diabetes is often characterized by two primary factors: insulin resistance and beta cell dysfunction. Insulin resistance occurs when the body's cells become less responsive to the effects of insulin, resulting in reduced glucose uptake. Concurrently, beta cells in the pancreas, responsible for producing insulin, may progressively lose their ability to meet the body's demand for this crucial hormone.

3. Risk Factors and Genetics

The risk factors for developing type 2 diabetes are diverse and multifaceted. While genetics can play a role, lifestyle factors exert significant influence. Family history, age, obesity, lack of physical activity, and poor dietary habits are among the key contributors. Understanding these risk factors is crucial for both prevention and management.

4. Symptoms of Type 2 Diabetes

Type 2 diabetes can manifest with a range of symptoms, although some individuals may remain asymptomatic, especially in the early stages. Common signs include increased thirst, frequent urination, unexplained weight loss, fatigue, blurred vision, and slow-healing wounds or infections. Recognizing these symptoms is pivotal for early diagnosis and intervention.

5. Diagnosis

The diagnosis of type 2 diabetes involves various blood tests that measure blood glucose levels. Fasting blood sugar tests and oral glucose tolerance tests are commonly employed to assess how the body handles glucose. Elevated blood sugar levels may prompt further diagnostic tests and a comprehensive evaluation by healthcare professionals.

6. Genetics and Lifestyle

While genetics can predispose individuals to type 2 diabetes, lifestyle factors play a significant role in its development. A sedentary lifestyle, poor dietary choices, and excess body weight, particularly abdominal obesity, are modifiable risk factors that contribute to insulin resistance and the onset of diabetes.

7. Prevalence and Global Impact

Type 2 diabetes has reached epidemic proportions globally, with a staggering rise in prevalence over the past few decades. The World Health Organization (WHO) estimates that over 400 million people live with diabetes, the majority of whom have type 2 diabetes. This prevalence is expected to rise further, making diabetes a major public health concern.

8. Impact on Health

Untreated or poorly managed type 2 diabetes can have profound consequences on various organ systems. The condition is associated with an increased risk of cardiovascular diseases, including heart attacks and strokes. Additionally, diabetes can lead to kidney damage, nerve damage (neuropathy), eye problems, and complications affecting the feet and skin.

9. Lifestyle Modification as a Cornerstone of Management

The cornerstone of type 2 diabetes management lies in lifestyle modifications. Adopting a healthy diet, engaging in regular physical activity, and maintaining a healthy weight are fundamental components. These changes aim to improve insulin sensitivity, regulate blood sugar levels, and mitigate the risk of complications.

10. Medications and Insulin Therapy

In some cases, lifestyle changes alone may not be sufficient to control blood sugar levels. Medications, ranging from oral drugs to injectable insulin, may be prescribed to complement lifestyle modifications. These medications work in various ways to enhance insulin action, reduce glucose production in the liver, or improve insulin secretion.

11. Blood Sugar Monitoring

Regular monitoring of blood sugar levels is a crucial aspect of diabetes management. Glucose meters allow individuals to measure their blood sugar levels at home, providing valuable information for adjusting diet, exercise, and medication as needed. Monitoring helps individuals and healthcare providers assess the effectiveness of the management plan.

12. Complications and Preventive Measures

Proactive management is essential to prevent or delay the onset of complications associated with type 2 diabetes. Routine medical check-ups, eye exams, and kidney function tests are integral components of preventive care. Blood pressure and cholesterol management also play crucial roles in reducing the risk of cardiovascular complications.

13. Psychosocial Aspects

Living with type 2 diabetes can impact mental and emotional well-being. The constant management, potential complications, and lifestyle adjustments can contribute to stress, anxiety, and depression. Recognizing and addressing these psychosocial aspects is integral to comprehensive diabetes care.

14. Empowerment and Education

Education is a powerful tool in the management of type 2 diabetes. Empowering individuals with knowledge about their condition, its management, and the importance of self-care fosters a sense of control. Support groups, educational resources, and healthcare provider guidance contribute to this ongoing process of empowerment.

15. Future Perspectives

Ongoing research in the field of diabetes continues to uncover new insights into the condition's complexities. Innovations in treatment modalities, advancements in monitoring technologies, and a deeper understanding of the genetic and environmental factors influencing type 2 diabetes offer hope for improved management and prevention strategies in the future.

Insulin Resistance and Beta Cell Dysfunction

Insulin resistance and beta cell dysfunction are two major components of type 2 diabetes. These two phenomena, which are part of the complex process of glucose regulation, provide insight into the intricate mechanisms that drive the development and progression of this common metabolic disorder. In this article, we will explore the molecular intricacies, the impact on overall health, diagnostic implications, and potential therapeutic interventions related to insulin resistance and beta cell dysfunction.

Understanding the Players: Insulin and Glucose Dynamics

Before we dive into the details of insulin resistance and beta cell dysfunction, it is important to understand the role of insulin in glucose regulation. Insulin, which is produced by the beta cells in the pancreas, acts like a key that unlocks cells to allow glucose entry. Glucose, which is derived from the digestion of carbohydrates in the diet, is a primary source of energy for cells. The delicate balance between insulin and glucose is essential for maintaining healthy blood sugar levels.

Insulin Resistance: Unraveling the Resistance Mechanism

Molecular Landscape

Insulin resistance is a condition in which the body's cells become less responsive to the effects of insulin, impairing the uptake of glucose. The exact mechanisms are complex, but they are linked to changes in signaling pathways and cellular responses. Intracellular pathways, such as the insulin receptor substrate (IRS) pathway, are disrupted, leading to decreased insulin sensitivity.

Adipose Tissue Dynamics

Adipose tissue, commonly known as fat, plays a major role in insulin resistance. Excessive fat accumulation, especially visceral adiposity (fat around organs), leads to the release of adipokines and inflammatory substances. These factors interfere with insulin signaling, creating an environment that promotes insulin resistance.

Muscle and Liver Involvement

Muscle and liver cells are the primary sites of glucose uptake. In insulin resistance, these cells become less responsive to insulin, impairing their ability to take up glucose. The liver, in particular, responds by increasing glucose production, further exacerbating elevated blood sugar levels.

Inflammation and Oxidative Stress

Chronic low-grade inflammation and oxidative stress are closely linked to insulin resistance. Inflammatory molecules, such as cytokines, and reactive oxygen species disrupt cellular signaling pathways, contributing to a state of insulin resistance. This inflammatory environment amplifies the metabolic dysfunction associated with type 2 diabetes.

Beta Cell Dysfunction: The Pancreatic Perspective

The Role of Beta Cells

Beta cells, located in the islets of Langerhans within the pancreas, are responsible for producing and releasing insulin in response to elevated blood glucose levels. These cells play a critical role in maintaining glucose homeostasis by adjusting insulin secretion based on the body's needs.

Challenges Faced by Beta Cells

In the context of type 2 diabetes, beta cells face several challenges. The prolonged demand for increased insulin secretion in response to insulin resistance can lead to a state of hyperfunction. Over time, this hyperfunction may lead to beta cell exhaustion and a decrease in their capacity to secrete insulin effectively.

Beta Cell Adaptations

Initially, beta cells attempt to compensate for insulin resistance by producing more insulin. This adaptive response, known as hyperinsulinemia, is an attempt to overcome the resistance and maintain glucose homeostasis. However, persistent demand can lead to a state where beta cells struggle to keep up with the escalating requirements.

Apoptosis and Dysfunction

As the demands on beta cells intensify, they may undergo apoptosis, a form of programmed cell death. This loss of beta cells contributes to reduced insulin secretion capacity. Additionally, dysfunctional beta cells may secrete insulin ineffectively, further complicating glucose regulation.

Influence of Genetic Factors

Genetic factors play a role in determining an individual's predisposition to beta cell dysfunction. Polymorphisms in genes associated with insulin secretion and beta cell function contribute to the variability in how individuals respond to insulin resistance.

Diagnostic Implications: Detecting the Underlying Dynamics

Blood Tests

Diagnosing insulin resistance and beta cell dysfunction often involves blood tests that measure various markers. Fasting insulin levels, combined with fasting glucose levels, can provide insights into insulin resistance. Additionally, tests measuring C-peptide, a byproduct of insulin production, offer information about beta cell function.

Oral Glucose Tolerance Test (OGTT)

The OGTT is a diagnostic tool that involves administering a standardized glucose solution and monitoring the body's response. This test provides a comprehensive view of how the body handles glucose, offering valuable information about both insulin resistance and beta cell function.

Hemoglobin A1c (HbA1c)

HbA1c is a test that measures the average blood sugar levels over the past two to three months. This test can be used to detect insulin resistance and beta cell dysfunction, as well as to monitor the effectiveness of therapeutic interventions.

Unraveling the Complexity of Type 2 Diabetes Risk Factors

Type 2 diabetes is a complex metabolic disorder that is influenced by a combination of genetic, lifestyle, and environmental factors. To better understand the various risk factors associated with this condition, it is essential to explore them in depth. In this comprehensive exploration, we will look at the diverse landscape of type 2 diabetes risk factors, from genetic predisposition to lifestyle choices and socio-economic determinants.

Genetic Predisposition: Unraveling the Genetic Tapestry

Family History

One of the most important risk factors for type 2 diabetes is a family history of the condition. People with close relatives, such as parents or siblings, who have diabetes are more likely to develop it. Genetic factors play a role in susceptibility, and certain gene variants can affect insulin production and glucose regulation.

Ethnicity and Genetics

The prevalence of type 2 diabetes varies among different ethnic groups, which emphasizes the role of genetic factors. For instance, individuals of African, Hispanic, Native American, and Asian descent are more likely to develop type 2 diabetes than those of European descent. Genetic research is continuing to uncover the specific mechanisms behind these ethnic disparities.

Genetic Polymorphisms

Specific genetic variations, known as polymorphisms, can influence an individual's susceptibility to type 2 diabetes. Polymorphisms in genes related to insulin secretion, insulin sensitivity, and glucose metabolism contribute to the heterogeneity in diabetes risk. Advances in genomic research are providing insights into these intricate genetic pathways.

Lifestyle Choices: The Power of Daily Decisions

Obesity: A Pervasive Risk

One of the most modifiable risk factors for type 2 diabetes is obesity. Excess body weight, particularly visceral adiposity (fat around internal organs), contributes to insulin resistance. Adipose tissue secretes inflammatory substances, creating an environment that is conducive to metabolic dysfunction. The rise in global obesity rates is linked to the increasing prevalence of type 2 diabetes.

Physical Inactivity: A Sedentary Culprit

A sedentary lifestyle is closely linked to the development of type 2 diabetes. Regular physical activity enhances insulin sensitivity, promotes glucose uptake by muscles, and helps maintain a healthy weight. On the other hand, a lack of exercise contributes to insulin resistance, obesity, and an increased risk of diabetes.

Dietary Choices: The Glucose Connection

Diet is a major factor in diabetes risk. Eating a diet high in refined carbohydrates, added sugars, and unhealthy fats can lead to insulin resistance and obesity. Conversely, a diet rich in whole grains, fruits, vegetables, and lean proteins supports glucose regulation and reduces diabetes risk.

Gestational Diabetes: A Window into Future Risk:

Women who experience gestational diabetes during pregnancy are more likely to develop type 2 diabetes later in life. This highlights the interconnectedness of reproductive health and metabolic outcomes, emphasizing the need for post-pregnancy monitoring and lifestyle interventions.

Metabolic Syndrome: A Cluster of Risk Factors

Defining Metabolic Syndrome:

Metabolic syndrome is a group of conditions that increase the risk of type 2 diabetes and cardiovascular disease. The components of metabolic syndrome include abdominal obesity, elevated blood pressure, high triglyceride levels, low HDL cholesterol, and impaired glucose tolerance. Having metabolic syndrome amplifies the overall risk profile for diabetes.

Insulin Resistance as a Common Thread:

Insulin resistance is a common factor in the components of metabolic syndrome. The impaired ability of cells to respond to insulin contributes to elevated blood sugar, dyslipidemia, and hypertension, creating a metabolic environment that is conducive to type 2 diabetes.

Age and Gender: Navigating the Demographic Landscape

Age as a Risk Modifier:

Age is a significant non-modifiable risk factor for type 2 diabetes. The risk increases with age, emphasizing the importance of preventive measures, especially in older populations. Aging is associated with changes in metabolism, body composition, and physical activity levels that contribute to diabetes risk.

Gender Disparities:

Gender influences diabetes risk, with variations in risk profiles between men and women. In the past, men were thought to be at a higher risk, but recent trends show a narrowing of this gender gap. Women with a history of gestational diabetes, polycystic ovary syndrome (PCOS), or a family history of diabetes may be more susceptible.

Socio-Economic Determinants: The Impact of Environment

Social Determinants of Health

Socio-economic status has a major influence on diabetes risk. People with lower socio-economic status may struggle to access healthy food, exercise regularly, and receive quality healthcare. This leads to a higher prevalence of diabetes in socio-economically disadvantaged populations.

Educational Attainment: Knowledge as a Shield

Education plays a role in forming health behaviors and access to resources. People with higher educational levels tend to have better health literacy, allowing them to make informed lifestyle choices. On the other hand, lower educational attainment is linked to an increased risk of diabetes.

Environmental Influences: Urbanization and Lifestyle Shifts

The environment in which people live, work, and play is a major factor in diabetes risk. Urbanization, sedentary jobs, and lifestyle changes create an obesogenic environment. Access to parks, recreational facilities, and healthy food options affects the choices people make regarding physical activity and diet.

Psychosocial Factors: The Mind-Body Connection

Chronic Stress: A Metabolic Disruptor:
Chronic stress can have a huge impact on metabolic health, leading to insulin resistance. The body's response to stress involves the release of hormones such as cortisol and adrenaline, which, when persistent, can cause glucose metabolism to become unbalanced.

Depression and Diabetes: A Bidirectional Relationship

The relationship between depression and type 2 diabetes is two-way. Depression can be both a risk factor for and a result of diabetes. Living with a chronic condition can take an emotional toll.

Decoding Type 2 Diabetes: Symptoms and Diagnosis Unveiled

Type 2 diabetes is a widespread and complex metabolic disorder that is characterized by high blood sugar levels, usually caused by insulin resistance and inadequate insulin production. Knowing the signs and diagnostic processes is essential for timely treatment and successful management. In this comprehensive overview, we will explore the subtle and obvious signs of type 2 diabetes and look into the diagnostic techniques that healthcare professionals use to confirm and monitor the condition.

The Range of Symptoms: Identifying the Clues

1. Polyuria (Excessive Urination):
   One of the main symptoms of type 2 diabetes is polyuria, or excessive urination. High blood sugar levels lead to increased urine production as the kidneys try to get rid of the extra glucose. People may find themselves making frequent trips to the restroom, especially at night (nocturia).

2. Polydipsia (Excessive Thirst):
   Excessive thirst, or polydipsia, is closely related to polyuria. As the body loses more fluids through increased urination, a persistent feeling of thirst follows. People may find themselves constantly reaching for fluids to quench their thirst.

3. Polyphagia (Excessive Hunger):
   Despite eating enough or more food, people with type 2 diabetes may experience persistent hunger or polyphagia. This paradoxical combination of increased hunger and weight loss can be attributed to the body's inability to effectively use glucose for energy.

4. Unexplained Weight Loss:
   Unintentional weight loss can be a warning sign of type 2 diabetes. Despite polyphagia, the body's inability to use glucose efficiently leads to the breakdown of muscle and fat for energy, resulting in weight loss.

5. Fatigue and Weakness:
   Chronic fatigue and weakness are common symptoms of type 2 diabetes. The body's inability to effectively use glucose leads to an energy deficit, causing feelings of fatigue even after adequate rest.

6. Blurred Vision:

Changes in vision, such as blurriness, can occur due to fluctuations in blood sugar levels. High glucose levels can lead to temporary changes in the shape of the lens of the eye, affecting focus.

7. Slow Wound Healing:

Impaired blood circulation and weakened immune system in people with type 2 diabetes can result in slow wound healing. Cuts and sores may take longer to heal, increasing the risk of infections.

8. Frequent Infections:

Reduced immune function associated with high blood sugar levels makes people with type 2 diabetes more prone to infections. Common sites for infections include the skin, urinary tract, and gums.

9. Tingling or Numbness (Peripheral Neuropathy):

High blood sugar levels can lead to nerve damage, particularly in the extremities. Tingling, numbness, or a burning sensation in the hands and feet may indicate peripheral neuropathy.

10.Itching and Skin Changes:

Dry skin, itching, and changes in skin texture can be associated with diabetes. Skin conditions such as acanthosis nigricans, characterized by dark, velvety patches, may also be observed.

Understanding the Diagnostic Landscape: Tools and Techniques

1. Fasting Blood Sugar Test:

The fasting blood sugar test is a basic diagnostic tool for identifying diabetes. It measures blood glucose levels after an overnight fast. A fasting blood sugar level of 126 milligrams per deciliter (mg/dL) or higher on two separate occasions indicates diabetes.

2. Oral Glucose Tolerance Test (OGTT):

The OGTT involves fasting overnight, followed by the consumption of a glucose solution. Blood sugar levels are then measured at intervals to assess the body's ability to process glucose. A two-hour blood sugar level of 200 mg/dL or higher indicates diabetes.

3. Hemoglobin A1c Test:

The hemoglobin A1c test provides an average of blood sugar levels over the past two to three months. An A1c level of 6.5% or higher is indicative of diabetes. This test is advantageous as it does not require fasting.

4. Random Blood Sugar Test:

A random blood sugar test measures glucose levels without regard to the time of the last meal. A blood sugar level of 200 mg/dL or higher, along with the presence of diabetes symptoms, may prompt further testing.

5. Glycated Albumin (GA) Test:

The glycated albumin test reflects average blood sugar levels over a shorter period than the A1c test. It may be used in situations where rapid changes in blood sugar are expected.

6. Continuous Glucose Monitoring (CGM):

CGM involves the use of a small sensor placed under the skin to measure glucose levels in real-time throughout the day and night. This data provides a comprehensive overview of glucose fluctuations.

7. C-peptide Test:

The C-peptide test measures the amount of C-peptide, a byproduct of insulin production. It helps to differentiate between type 1 and type 2 diabetes and assesses the body's insulin production.

8. Urinalysis:

Urinalysis may be conducted to detect the presence of ketones or excess glucose in the urine, which can indicate poor blood sugar control. It is particularly useful in diagnosing and monitoring diabetes in certain situations.

9. Screening for Complications:

In addition to glucose-focused tests, healthcare professionals may conduct screenings for diabetes-related complications. These may include eye exams to check for diabetic retinopathy, kidney function tests, and nerve function tests.

Challenges in Diagnosis: The Nuances of Early Detection

1. Asymptomatic Nature:

   In the early stages, type 2 diabetes may be asymptomatic, leading to delayed diagnosis. Regular health check-ups and screenings for individuals with risk factors are essential for early detection.

2. Insidious Onset:

   The gradual onset of symptoms may be overlooked or attributed to other factors, causing people to underestimate the significance of their symptoms.

3. Overlap with Other Conditions:

   Symptoms of type 2 diabetes, such as fatigue and frequent urination, can be similar to those of other health conditions. This makes it important for healthcare professionals to consider a comprehensive clinical picture.

4. Risk-Based Screening:

   Identifying individuals at risk through risk-based screening strategies is essential for early detection. Risk factors, including family history, obesity, age, and ethnic background, guide targeted screening efforts.

The Role of Healthcare Professionals: Collaborative Care and Education

1. Primary Care Physicians:

Primary care physicians play a major role in the early detection and management of type 2 diabetes. Routine health check-ups, monitoring of risk factors, and prompt referral for diagnostic tests are important for timely intervention.

2. Endocrinologists:

Endocrinologists, specialists in hormonal disorders, are key members of the healthcare team for individuals with diabetes. They provide expertise in diabetes management, especially in cases requiring advanced treatment strategies.

3. Diabetes Educators:

Diabetes educators are essential in giving individuals the knowledge and skills needed to manage their condition. They offer guidance on lifestyle modifications, medication adherence, blood sugar monitoring, and overall self-care.

4. Nutritionists and Dietitians:

Nutritionists and dietitians are important partners in diabetes care. They help individuals create personalized meal plans that align with their dietary preferences and health goals. A balanced and nutrient-rich diet is essential for managing blood sugar levels and overall well-being.

5. Nurse Practitioners and Physician Assistants:

Nurse practitioners and physician assistants often work closely with primary care physicians and endocrinologists in diabetes management. They provide ongoing support, assist with medication management, and educate individuals on various aspects of diabetes care.

6. Pharmacists:

Pharmacists are valuable resources for individuals with diabetes, providing information on medications, potential side effects, and ensuring proper medication adherence. They play a role in medication management and may offer insights on over-the-counter medications and supplements.

7. Mental Health Professionals

Mental health professionals, including psychologists and counselors, contribute to holistic diabetes care by addressing the psychological and emotional aspects of living with a chronic condition. They help individuals cope with stress, anxiety, and depression that may be associated with diabetes.

8. Ongoing Monitoring and Follow-up:

Diabetes management is a dynamic process that requires ongoing monitoring and follow-up. Regular check-ups, blood tests, and assessments of complications risk are essential components of comprehensive diabetes care.

The Importance of Patient Engagement: Empowering Individuals

1. Health Literacy:

Health literacy is essential for individuals to understand their condition, treatment options, and the importance of self-management. Effective communication between healthcare providers and patients is necessary for informed decision-making.

2. Self-Monitoring:

Self-monitoring of blood sugar levels, diet, physical activity, and other relevant parameters empowers individuals to take part in their diabetes care. It provides valuable insights and allows for timely adjustments to the management plan.

3. Lifestyle Modifications:

Lifestyle modifications, including dietary changes, regular physical activity, and weight management, are foundational elements of diabetes care. Empowering individuals to adopt and sustain these modifications contributes to overall well-being.

4. Medication Adherence:

Adherence to prescribed medications is crucial for effective diabetes management. Educating individuals about the purpose, dosage, and potential side effects of medications enhances adherence and optimizes treatment outcomes.

5. Problem-Solving Skills:

Developing problem-solving skills equips individuals to navigate challenges associated with diabetes management. This includes addressing fluctuations in blood sugar levels, understanding the impact of lifestyle choices, and seeking timely support when needed.

6. Regular Follow-up:

Regular follow-up with healthcare providers ensures ongoing monitoring of blood sugar levels, adjustments to the treatment plan as needed, and proactive management of potential complications. It establishes a collaborative approach to long-term diabetes care.

7. Support Networks:

Building a support network, whether through family, friends, or diabetes support groups, provides emotional support and a sense of community. Sharing experiences, tips, and coping strategies fosters a supportive environment for individuals with diabetes.

Chapter 2: The Impact of Lifestyle on Type 2 Diabetes

Type 2 diabetes is a chronic metabolic condition that is heavily influenced by lifestyle choices. In this exploration, we will explore the intricate connections between lifestyle and type 2 diabetes, focusing on the impact of diet, physical activity, weight management, and other lifestyle components on this prevalent health condition.

Dietary Choices: The Foundation of Metabolic Health

1. Carbohydrate Quality and Quantity:

   The type and amount of carbohydrates consumed can have a major impact on blood sugar levels. Eating a lot of refined carbohydrates and added sugars can cause rapid spikes in blood glucose, leading to insulin resistance. On the other hand, consuming whole grains, fruits, vegetables, and legumes can help keep blood sugar levels stable and promote overall metabolic health.

2. Protein and Healthy Fats:

   Including lean protein sources and healthy fats in the diet can help with satiety, stabilize blood sugar, and support weight management. Healthy fats, such as those found in avocados, nuts, and olive oil, have been linked to improved insulin sensitivity.

3. Portion Control:

   Portion control is essential for managing caloric intake and blood sugar levels. Overeating, even of nutritious foods, can lead to weight gain and insulin resistance. Being mindful of portion sizes and practicing intuitive eating can help create a balanced and sustainable approach to nutrition.

4. Meal Timing:

   The timing of meals can have an effect on blood sugar regulation. Eating meals throughout the day and avoiding long periods of fasting can help prevent large fluctuations in blood glucose levels. Consistent meal timing can also support the body's natural circadian rhythm.

5. Nutrient Density:

Choosing nutrient-dense foods provides essential vitamins, minerals, and antioxidants that support overall health. Nutrient-dense options include a variety of colorful fruits and vegetables, whole grains, and lean protein sources.

Physical Activity: Empowering the Body and Mind

1. Insulin Sensitivity and Exercise:

Regular physical activity can increase insulin sensitivity, allowing cells to more effectively use glucose. Exercise stimulates the uptake of glucose by muscles, reducing the need for insulin for glucose transport.

2. Cardiovascular Exercise:

Cardiovascular exercises, such as walking, jogging, swimming, and cycling, can help with weight management and cardiovascular health. These activities improve blood circulation, reduce blood pressure, and have a positive effect on lipid profiles.

3. Strength Training:

Incorporating strength training into an exercise routine can help build lean muscle mass. Muscle tissue is more metabolically active, aiding in glucose uptake and contributing to improved insulin sensitivity.

4. Flexibility and Balance:

Activities that enhance flexibility and balance, such as yoga and tai chi, can contribute to overall well-being. They can promote relaxation, reduce stress, and may have a positive effect on insulin sensitivity.

5. Consistency is Key:

Consistency in physical activity is essential for long-term benefits. Developing a routine that includes a combination of aerobic, strength, and flexibility exercises can help promote sustainable health outcomes.

Weight Management: Balancing the Equation

1. Body Mass Index (BMI) and Diabetes Risk:

Keeping a healthy weight is key for type 2 diabetes prevention and management. Excess body weight, especially visceral fat, can lead to insulin resistance. Monitoring body mass index (BMI) can help assess the relationship between weight and diabetes risk.

2. Weight Loss Strategies:

For people with overweight or obesity, intentional weight loss can result in significant improvements in insulin sensitivity. Lifestyle modifications, such as dietary changes and increased physical activity, are effective strategies for sustainable weight management.

3. Waist Circumference:

Waist circumference is a useful indicator of abdominal obesity, which is particularly linked to insulin resistance. Reducing waist circumference through lifestyle changes can help improve metabolic health.

Sleep Quality and Stress Management: Balancing the Equation

1. Sleep and Hormonal Regulation:

Adequate and quality sleep is connected to hormonal regulation, including insulin. Sleep deprivation can disrupt the balance of hormones that affect hunger, satiety, and glucose metabolism, leading to insulin resistance.

2. Stress and Cortisol Levels:

Chronic stress can raise cortisol levels, which can interfere with insulin sensitivity. Stress management techniques, such as mindfulness, meditation, and relaxation exercises, can help create a more balanced hormonal environment.

3. Smoking and Alcohol Consumption:

Smoking and excessive alcohol consumption are associated with an increased risk of type 2 diabetes. Quitting smoking and moderating alcohol intake can have a positive effect on overall health and contribute to better metabolic health.

The intricate relationship between obesity and Type 2 diabetes is undeniable, with obesity being a major factor in this complex connection. Excess body weight, particularly in the form of visceral fat, has a significant impact on the risk, progression, and management of Type 2 diabetes. In this discussion, we will explore the intricate relationship between obesity and Type 2 diabetes, looking at the physiological mechanisms, risk factors, and the essential role of lifestyle interventions in breaking this link.

Understanding the Physiology: How Obesity Drives Insulin Resistance

1. Adipose Tissue as an Endocrine Organ:

Adipose tissue, commonly known as fat, is not just a storage site for excess calories; it is an endocrine organ. In obesity, adipose tissue undergoes structural and functional changes, releasing pro-inflammatory cytokines, adipokines, and free fatty acids. These substances create a chronic low-grade inflammatory state that contributes to insulin resistance.

2. Insulin Resistance: The Key Precursor:

Insulin resistance, a hallmark of Type 2 diabetes, occurs when cells fail to respond effectively to insulin's signal. In obesity, adipose tissue-derived factors interfere with insulin signaling pathways. As a result, cells, particularly in the muscles and liver, become less responsive to insulin, leading to elevated blood glucose levels.

3. Inflammatory Response:

Chronic inflammation induced by obesity exacerbates insulin resistance. Inflammatory mediators, such as tumor necrosis factor-alpha (TNF-α) and interleukin-6 (IL-6), disrupt insulin signaling pathways and contribute to the dysfunction of insulin-responsive tissues.

4. Ectopic Fat Accumulation:

Obesity often results in ectopic fat accumulation, where fat is deposited in organs like the liver and pancreas. In the liver, excessive fat leads to increased production of glucose, contributing to hyperglycemia. In the pancreas, fat accumulation may impair beta cell function, diminishing insulin secretion.

The Obesity-Diabetes Link: Unraveling Risk Factors

1. Central Obesity: A Strong Predictor:

Central obesity, characterized by an excess of abdominal fat, is a strong predictor of Type 2 diabetes risk. Visceral fat, located around internal organs, is metabolically active and releases substances that promote insulin resistance.

2. Body Mass Index (BMI):

Body Mass Index (BMI), a measure of body fat based on height and weight, is commonly used to assess obesity. Individuals with a BMI in the overweight or obese range are at an increased risk of developing Type 2 diabetes.

3. Waist-to-Hip Ratio:

Waist-to-hip ratio, a measure of body fat distribution, provides insights into central obesity. A higher ratio indicates a greater concentration of abdominal fat, elevating the risk of insulin resistance and Type 2 diabetes.

4. Genetic Factors:

Genetic factors play a role in determining an individual's susceptibility to both obesity and Type 2 diabetes. Shared genetic predispositions contribute to the clustering of these conditions within families.

5. Lifestyle Factors:

Unhealthy lifestyle choices, such as a sedentary lifestyle and poor dietary habits, contribute to both obesity and Type 2 diabetes. Physical inactivity and excessive caloric intake, especially from refined carbohydrates and added sugars, fuel the obesity-diabetes connection.

Breaking the Link: Lifestyle Interventions for Diabetes Prevention

The importance of lifestyle interventions in preventing and managing Type 2 diabetes cannot be overstated. Diabetes education programs provide individuals with the knowledge and skills needed to make informed lifestyle choices. Additionally, building a support network, whether through healthcare professionals, family, friends, or diabetes support groups, fosters a sense of community. Breaking up sitting time with short bouts of physical activity and reducing screen time, especially before bedtime, can also help mitigate the negative effects of sedentary behavior. By making healthy lifestyle choices, individuals can empower themselves to break the link between obesity and Type 2 diabetes.

1. Weight Loss and Improved Insulin Sensitivity

Weight loss is a cornerstone in the management and prevention of Type 2 diabetes. Even modest weight loss has been shown to improve insulin sensitivity, leading to better blood glucose control. Lifestyle interventions that incorporate a balanced diet and increased physical activity are central to achieving sustainable weight loss.

2. Physical Activity: A Powerful Ally

Regular physical activity plays a crucial role in preventing and managing Type 2 diabetes, especially in the context of obesity. Exercise enhances insulin sensitivity, promotes weight loss, and helps regulate blood glucose levels. Both aerobic exercises and strength training contribute to overall metabolic health.

3. Dietary Modifications

Adopting a healthy and balanced diet is fundamental in addressing both obesity and Type 2 diabetes. Emphasizing whole foods, such as fruits, vegetables, whole grains, and lean proteins, while minimizing processed foods and added sugars, supports weight management and improves insulin sensitivity.

4. Behavioral Changes

Behavioral modifications, including adopting mindful eating practices and addressing emotional eating, contribute to sustainable lifestyle changes. Behavioral interventions aim to reshape habits and foster a positive relationship with food, promoting long-term well-being.

5. Bariatric Surgery

For individuals with severe obesity and Type 2 diabetes, bariatric surgery may be considered. Weight loss surgeries, such as gastric bypass or sleeve gastrectomy, often lead to significant improvements in insulin sensitivity and diabetes remission.

The Role of Healthcare Professionals: Collaborative Care for Holistic Wellness

1. Multidisciplinary Approach

The management of obesity and Type 2 diabetes requires a multidisciplinary approach. Healthcare professionals, including physicians, dietitians, physical therapists, and behavioral therapists, collaborate to address the diverse aspects of these interconnected conditions.

2. Personalized Care Plans:

Personalized care plans, tailored to individual needs and preferences, enhance the effectiveness of interventions. Understanding the unique factors influencing a person's obesity and diabetes allows for targeted and sustainable strategies.

3. Continuous Monitoring and Support

Ongoing monitoring of weight, blood glucose levels, and overall health is essential for long-term success. Continuous support from healthcare professionals fosters accountability and enables individuals to navigate challenges effectively.
 Importance of regular physical activity

Regular physical activity stands as a cornerstone in the comprehensive management of Type 2 diabetes, offering a multitude of benefits that extend far beyond the realm of cardiovascular fitness. For individuals living with Type 2 diabetes, integrating regular exercise into their routine is a powerful tool for enhancing insulin sensitivity, controlling blood sugar levels, and improving overall well-being. In this exploration, we delve into the significance of regular physical activity in the context of Type 2 diabetes, examining its impact on metabolic health, cardiovascular function, and the broader spectrum of diabetes management.

Enhancing Insulin Sensitivity: A Key Mechanism

1. Improved Glucose Uptake:
 Regular physical activity enhances the body's ability to utilize glucose by increasing insulin sensitivity. As muscles contract during exercise, they facilitate the uptake of glucose, reducing reliance on insulin for glucose transport. This process contributes to better blood sugar control.

2. Muscle Glucose Metabolism:
 Physical activity stimulates the muscles to efficiently metabolize glucose. This effect is particularly significant for individuals with insulin resistance, as exercise helps overcome the impaired responsiveness of cells to insulin.

3. Mitigating Insulin Resistance:
 Insulin resistance, a hallmark of Type 2 diabetes, is mitigated through regular physical activity. Exercise promotes changes at the cellular level, enhancing insulin signaling pathways and fostering a more responsive cellular environment.

Blood Sugar Control: Balancing the Glucose Equation

1. Post-Exercise Glucose Utilization:

The benefits of exercise extend beyond the immediate activity period. Post-exercise, the body continues to utilize glucose effectively, leading to a sustained reduction in blood sugar levels. This effect is particularly valuable for individuals with diabetes who experience fluctuations in blood glucose.

2. Improved A1c Levels:

A1c, or hemoglobin A1c, is a marker that reflects average blood sugar levels over the past two to three months. Regular physical activity contributes to improved A1c levels, providing a measure of long-term glycemic control.

3. Preventing Hyperglycemia:

Physical activity helps prevent hyperglycemia, the condition characterized by excessively high blood sugar levels. By enhancing insulin sensitivity and glucose utilization, exercise acts as a natural safeguard against spikes in blood glucose.

Cardiovascular Health: Strengthening the Heart

1. Reducing Cardiovascular Risk:

Individuals with Type 2 diabetes face an increased risk of cardiovascular complications. Regular physical activity helps mitigate this risk by improving cardiovascular health. It lowers blood pressure, reduces cholesterol levels, and supports overall heart function.

2. Enhanced Circulation:

Exercise enhances blood circulation, ensuring that vital organs, including the heart, receive an adequate supply of oxygen and nutrients. Improved circulation contributes to the prevention of vascular complications associated with diabetes.

3. Weight Management: A Dual Benefit:

Physical activity is integral to weight management, which is crucial for cardiovascular health in individuals with Type 2 diabetes. Maintaining a healthy weight reduces the strain on the heart and decreases the risk of obesity-related cardiovascular conditions.

Comprehensive Diabetes Management: Beyond Glucose Control

1. Weight Maintenance and Loss:

Regular physical activity plays a central role in weight maintenance and loss. For individuals with Type 2 diabetes, achieving and maintaining a healthy weight is vital for overall metabolic health. Exercise contributes to caloric expenditure, supporting weight management goals.

2. Enhanced Mood and Mental Health:

Exercise is a powerful mood regulator and stress reducer. Individuals with Type 2 diabetes often face the challenges of managing a chronic condition, and regular physical activity provides an outlet for stress, anxiety, and depression. The mental health benefits contribute to a holistic approach to diabetes management.

3. Improved Sleep Patterns:

Quality sleep is crucial for individuals with Type 2 diabetes, as it influences glucose metabolism and hormonal regulation. Regular exercise contributes to improved sleep patterns, fostering better overall health and diabetes management.

Guidelines and Considerations for Physical Activity in Type 2 Diabetes

1. Individualized Approach:

Physical activity recommendations should be tailored to individual capabilities, preferences, and health status. An individualized approach ensures that the exercise plan aligns with the person's unique needs and accommodates any existing health conditions.

2. Combination of Aerobic and Strength Training:

A well-rounded exercise routine for individuals with Type 2 diabetes should include both aerobic exercises (such as brisk walking, cycling, or swimming) and strength training. Aerobic activities enhance cardiovascular fitness, while strength training supports muscle health and metabolism.

3. Consistency

Consistency in physical activity is paramount. Regular, sustained exercise yields the most significant benefits for glycemic control, cardiovascular health, and overall well-being. Establishing a routine and incorporating physical activity into daily life fosters a habit that contributes to long-term success.

4. Consultation with Healthcare Professionals:

Before initiating an exercise regimen, individuals with Type 2 diabetes should consult with their healthcare team. This ensures that the chosen activities align with their health status, medications, and specific diabetes management goals.

Chapter 3: Crafting Your 30-Day Meal Plan

In this chapter, we'll be taking a journey to create a personalized 30-day meal plan that is tailored to individuals with Type 2 diabetes. We understand the importance of nutrition in diabetes management, so this chapter will serve as a practical guide to help you make informed and nourishing choices that will help you maintain stable blood sugar levels and overall well-being.

Section 1: Understanding Nutritional Foundations

1. Balancing Macronutrients:
   Learn how to balance macronutrients—carbohydrates, proteins, and fats—in your daily meals. Knowing the impact of each macronutrient on blood sugar levels will give you the power to create meals that will help you maintain optimal glucose control.

2. Fiber-Rich Choices:
   Discover the world of fiber-rich foods, such as whole grains, fruits, and vegetables. Fiber not only aids in digestion but also helps regulate blood sugar levels by slowing the absorption of glucose.

3. Mindful Carbohydrate Choices:
   Dive into the details of carbohydrate choices, distinguishing between complex carbohydrates and refined sugars. Crafting a meal plan that focuses on whole, unprocessed carbohydrates will give you sustained energy and better glycemic control.

Section 2: Building Your Meal Plan

1. Breakfast Delights:
   Begin your day with a variety of nutritious and satisfying breakfast options. From hearty whole-grain cereals to protein-packed omelet with colorful vegetables, find choices that will fuel your morning without causing blood sugar spikes.

2. Lunchtime Staples:
   Explore a range of lunchtime staples that will give you the right balance of nutrients. From vibrant salads with lean proteins to whole-grain wraps filled with nutrient-rich ingredients, find options that will keep you energized throughout the day.

3. Dinner Creations:

Learn the art of crafting balanced and flavorful dinners. From grilled salmon with roasted vegetables to quinoa-stuffed bell peppers, discover dinner options that prioritize both taste and nutrition.

4. Snacking with Purpose:

Embrace the concept of mindful snacking by incorporating nutrient-dense choices into your daily routine. From Greek yogurt with berries to a handful of mixed nuts, find snacks that will satisfy cravings without compromising your health goals.

5. Hydration Strategies:

Explore the importance of hydration in diabetes management. Discover creative ways to stay well-hydrated, such as infused water with citrus and herbs, and understand how proper hydration supports overall health.

Section 3: Meal Planning Strategies

1. Batch Cooking and Meal Prep:

Learn the art of batch cooking and meal prepping to make your 30-day meal plan easier. Discover how preparing ingredients in advance can save time and make sure you always have wholesome options readily available.

2. Portion Control Techniques:

Understand the significance of portion control in diabetes management. Uncover practical techniques for managing portion sizes to avoid overeating and promote steady blood sugar levels.

3. Glycemic Index Awareness:

Get to know the glycemic index and its role in meal planning. Learn how to choose foods with lower glycemic indices to minimize post-meal blood sugar fluctuations.

Section 4: Culinary Creativity and Flavorful Options

1. **Herbs and Spices for Flavor:

Explore the world of herbs and spices to add flavor to your meals without relying on excess salt or sugar. Discover how culinary creativity can transform your dishes into delicious and diabetes-friendly culinary delights.

2. Cuisine Variety:

Enjoy the richness of global cuisines while adhering to your diabetes-friendly meal plan. From Mediterranean-inspired dishes to Asian-infused flavors, diversify your palate while managing blood sugar effectively.

3. Sweet Treats with a Twist:

Indulge your sweet tooth with diabetes-friendly dessert options. From fruit-based delights to recipes using natural sweeteners, learn how to enjoy treats without compromising your health goals.

Section 5: Navigating Dining Out and Social Situations

1. Smart Choices at Restaurants:

Navigate restaurant menus with confidence by understanding how to make smart and diabetes-friendly choices. From choosing lean proteins to opting for side dishes rich in fiber, master the art of dining out while managing blood sugar.

2. Socializing with Health in Mind

Approach social situations with a focus on health. Learn how to make informed choices at gatherings, parties, and events, so you can enjoy the company of others while still maintaining your diabetes management goals.

The Importance of a Balanced Diet: A Guide

Blood Sugar Regulation: The Core Objective

1. Impact on Glycemic Control:

Eating a balanced diet is essential for regulating blood sugar levels, a major concern for those with Type 2 diabetes. Choosing the right carbohydrates, such as whole grains, legumes, fruits, and vegetables, helps prevent sudden spikes and drops in blood glucose.

2. Balancing Macronutrients:

Achieving the right balance of macronutrients—carbohydrates, proteins, and fats—ensures a steady release of glucose into the bloodstream. This balance supports insulin function, allowing cells to use glucose effectively.

3. Portion Control:

Monitoring portion sizes is key to avoiding overconsumption of carbohydrates, which can lead to high blood sugar levels. Controlling portion sizes also helps with weight management, another important aspect of Type 2 diabetes care.

Weight Management: A Dual Benefit

1. Preventing and Managing Obesity

Weight management is closely linked to Type 2 diabetes, as excess body weight can lead to insulin resistance. A balanced diet helps with weight control by providing nutrient-dense foods that satisfy hunger without excess calories.

2. Promoting Healthy Body Composition:

Eating a balanced diet encourages the maintenance of lean muscle mass while reducing excess fat. This composition is associated with improved insulin sensitivity and better overall metabolic health.

Cardiovascular Health: Mitigating Risks

1. Controlling Cholesterol Levels:

People with Type 2 diabetes often face an increased risk of cardiovascular complications. A balanced diet, low in saturated and trans fats, helps control cholesterol levels, reducing the risk of heart disease and stroke.

2. Managing Blood Pressure:

Sodium intake, often associated with processed and high-sodium foods, can affect blood pressure. A balanced diet that includes whole, unprocessed foods helps regulate sodium levels, contributing to better blood pressure control.

Nutrient Density and Micronutrients:

1. Ensuring Essential Nutrients:

A balanced diet provides essential vitamins and minerals necessary for overall health. These micronutrients contribute to various bodily functions, including immune system support, bone health, and antioxidant protection.

2. Reducing Inflammation:

Chronic inflammation is associated with insulin resistance and other complications of Type 2 diabetes. Nutrient-dense foods with anti-inflammatory properties, such as fruits, vegetables, and omega-3 fatty acids, help reduce inflammation.

Gut Health: A Holistic Approach

1. Fiber-Rich Choices:

Including fiber-rich foods in a balanced diet promotes gut health. Fiber supports digestive regularity, aids in nutrient absorption, and may contribute to a healthier gut microbiome.

2. Preventing Digestive Issues:

Maintaining a balance of soluble and insoluble fiber can help prevent common digestive issues, such as constipation, which individuals with Type 2 diabetes may be more prone to experience.

Individualization and Sustainability:

1. Tailored to Personal Needs:

A balanced diet is not a one-size-fits-all approach. It can be tailored to individual preferences, cultural considerations, and dietary restrictions, making it a sustainable and realistic choice for long-term adherence.

2. Culinary Variety:

Eating a balanced diet doesn't mean sacrificing culinary enjoyment. It encourages a diverse range of foods, flavors, and cooking methods, fostering a positive and satisfying relationship with food.

Educational Empowerment:

1. Nutrition Education:
Knowing the principles of a balanced diet empowers individuals with Type 2 diabetes to make informed choices. Nutrition education is a key part of self-management, allowing individuals to confidently navigate food choices.

2. Incorporating Practical Knowledge:
Practical knowledge about food labels, portion control, and meal planning empowers individuals to make daily choices that align with their health goals and contribute to effective Type 2 diabetes management.

The Importance of a Balanced Diet: A Guide

Blood Sugar Regulation: The Core Objective

1. Impact on Glycemic Control:
Eating a balanced diet is essential for regulating blood sugar levels, a major concern for those with Type 2 diabetes. Choosing the right carbohydrates, such as whole grains, legumes, fruits, and vegetables, helps prevent sudden spikes and drops in blood glucose.

2. Balancing Macronutrients:
Achieving the right balance of macronutrients—carbohydrates, proteins, and fats—ensures a steady release of glucose into the bloodstream. This balance supports insulin function, allowing cells to use glucose effectively.

3. Portion Control:
Monitoring portion sizes is key to avoiding overconsumption of carbohydrates, which can lead to high blood sugar levels. Controlling portion sizes also helps with weight management, another important aspect of Type 2 diabetes care.

Weight Management: A Dual Benefit

1. Preventing and Managing Obesity
Weight management is closely linked to Type 2 diabetes, as excess body weight can lead to insulin resistance. A balanced diet helps with weight control by providing nutrient-dense foods that satisfy hunger without excess calories.

2. Promoting Healthy Body Composition:
Eating a balanced diet encourages the maintenance of lean muscle mass while reducing excess fat. This composition is associated with improved insulin sensitivity and better overall metabolic health.

Cardiovascular Health: Mitigating Risks

1. Controlling Cholesterol Levels:
People with Type 2 diabetes often face an increased risk of cardiovascular complications. A balanced diet, low in saturated and trans fats, helps control cholesterol levels, reducing the risk of heart disease and stroke.

2. Managing Blood Pressure:

Sodium intake, often associated with processed and high-sodium foods, can affect blood pressure. A balanced diet that includes whole, unprocessed foods helps regulate sodium levels, contributing to better blood pressure control.

Nutrient Density and Micronutrients:

1. Ensuring Essential Nutrients:

A balanced diet provides essential vitamins and minerals necessary for overall health. These micronutrients contribute to various bodily functions, including immune system support, bone health, and antioxidant protection.

2. Reducing Inflammation:

Chronic inflammation is associated with insulin resistance and other complications of Type 2 diabetes. Nutrient-dense foods with anti-inflammatory properties, such as fruits, vegetables, and omega-3 fatty acids, help reduce inflammation.

Gut Health: A Holistic Approach

1. Fiber-Rich Choices:

Including fiber-rich foods in a balanced diet promotes gut health. Fiber supports digestive regularity, aids in nutrient absorption, and may contribute to a healthier gut microbiome.

2. Preventing Digestive Issues:

Maintaining a balance of soluble and insoluble fiber can help prevent common digestive issues, such as constipation, which individuals with Type 2 diabetes may be more prone to experience.

Individualization and Sustainability:

1. Tailored to Personal Needs:

A balanced diet is not a one-size-fits-all approach. It can be tailored to individual preferences, cultural considerations, and dietary restrictions, making it a sustainable and realistic choice for long-term adherence.

2. Culinary Variety:

Eating a balanced diet doesn't mean sacrificing culinary enjoyment. It encourages a diverse range of foods, flavors, and cooking methods, fostering a positive and satisfying relationship with food.

Educational Empowerment:

1. Nutrition Education:

Knowing the principles of a balanced diet empowers individuals with Type 2 diabetes to make informed choices. Nutrition education is a key part of self-management, allowing individuals to confidently navigate food choices.

2. Incorporating Practical Knowledge:

Practical knowledge about food labels, portion control, and meal planning empowers individuals to make daily choices that align with their health goals and contribute to effective Type 2 diabetes management.

Guidelines For Meal Planning

Meal planning is an essential part of managing Type 2 diabetes, as it helps individuals make informed and intentional choices that can help regulate blood sugar levels, maintain a healthy weight, and promote overall well-being. To help you get started, here are some guidelines to consider when creating a meal plan tailored to your needs:

1. Balance Macronutrients: Focus on complex carbohydrates from whole grains, legumes, fruits, and vegetables, and monitor portion sizes to manage blood sugar levels. Include lean protein sources such as poultry, fish, tofu, legumes, and low-fat dairy, and choose healthy fats like avocados, nuts, seeds, and olive oil. Limit saturated and trans fats found in processed and fried foods.

2. Watch Portion Sizes: Be mindful of portion control to avoid overeating and stabilize blood sugar levels. Use smaller plates and bowls to help control portion sizes visually, and consider measuring food initially to develop an understanding of appropriate portions.

3. Emphasize Fiber-Rich Foods: Incorporate high-fiber foods like whole grains, fruits, vegetables, legumes, and nuts. Fiber helps regulate blood sugar, supports digestive health, and contributes to a feeling of fullness.

4. Choose Low-Glycemic Foods: Select foods with a low glycemic index (GI) to minimize post-meal blood sugar spikes. Low-GI foods include whole grains, non-starchy vegetables, and most fruits in moderation.

5. Include Lean Proteins: Opt for lean protein sources to support muscle health and satiety. Examples include poultry, fish, tofu, legumes, and low-fat dairy products.

6. Prioritize Whole, Unprocessed Foods: Choose whole, unprocessed foods over refined and processed options. Whole foods provide essential nutrients and are generally lower in added sugars and unhealthy fats.

7. Limit Added Sugars: Be aware of added sugars in foods and beverages, as they can contribute to blood sugar spikes. Read food labels to identify hidden sources of added sugars.

8. Monitor Sodium Intake: Limit sodium intake to support cardiovascular health. Choose fresh, whole foods over processed and packaged items, and use herbs and spices for flavor.

9. Stay Hydrated: Drink plenty of water throughout the day to stay hydrated. Limit sugary drinks and opt for water, herbal tea, or other low-calorie beverages.

10. Plan Regular, Balanced Meals: Aim for regular meal times to help regulate blood sugar levels. Include a mix of carbohydrates, proteins, and fats in each meal to provide sustained energy.

11. Consider Meal Timing: Distribute carbohydrate intake evenly throughout the day to avoid large spikes in blood sugar. Pay attention to how different foods affect blood sugar at different times of the day.

12. Individualize Your Plan: Work with a healthcare professional or registered dietitian to create a personalized meal plan based on your specific health needs, preferences, and lifestyle. Consider factors such as age, activity level, medications, and personal preferences when planning meals.

13. Monitor Blood Sugar Levels: Regularly monitor blood sugar levels as advised by healthcare professionals to understand the impact of different foods on your body. Use this information to make adjustments to your meal plan as needed.

14. Plan for Flexibility: Allow for flexibility in your meal plan to accommodate different situations and unexpected events. Learn how to make healthier choices when dining out or facing unexpected changes in your routine.

15. Seek Professional Guidance: Consult with a healthcare team, including a registered dietitian or nutritionist, to receive personalized guidance and ongoing support in managing Type 2 diabetes through nutrition.

Sample Grocery List

Creating a grocery list for managing Type 2 diabetes requires selecting nutrient-dense foods while keeping portion sizes and dietary goals in mind. Here's a sample grocery list that includes a variety of food categories:

Proteins:
- Skinless chicken breasts or thighs
- Salmon or other fatty fish (rich in omega-3 fatty acids)
- Lean ground turkey or chicken
- Eggs
- Greek yogurt (unsweetened, low-fat)
- Tofu or tempeh
- Canned beans (kidney beans, black beans, chickpeas)

Vegetables:
- Broccoli
- Spinach or kale
- Bell peppers (variety of colors)
- Cauliflower
- Zucchini or yellow squash
- Tomatoes
- Leafy greens (lettuce, arugula)

Fruits:
- Berries (strawberries, blueberries, raspberries)
- Apples
- Oranges or mandarins
- Avocado
- Lemons or limes
- Bananas (in moderation)
- Grapes

Whole Grains:
- Quinoa
- Brown rice
- Whole wheat pasta or brown rice noodles

- Oats (steel-cut or rolled)
- Whole grain bread or wraps
- Barley or bulgur

Legumes:
- Lentils
- Black beans
- Chickpeas
- Edamame

Dairy or Dairy Alternatives:
- Low-fat or skim milk
- Greek yogurt (unsweetened)
- Cottage cheese (low-fat)
- Cheese (in moderation)
- Almond or soy milk (unsweetened)

Nuts and Seeds:
- Almonds
- Walnuts
- Chia seeds
- Flaxseeds
- Pumpkin seeds

Healthy Fats:
- Olive oil
- Avocado oil
- Avocado
- Nuts and seeds

Herbs and Spices:
- Garlic
- Ginger
- Basil
- Cilantro
- Rosemary
- Cinnamon

- Turmeric

Condiments and Sauces:
- Tomato sauce (no added sugar)
- Mustard
- Vinegar (balsamic, apple cider)
- Low-sodium soy sauce
- Salsa (fresh or jarred)
- Hot sauce (if preferred)

Beverages:
- Water
- Herbal tea (unsweetened)
- Sparkling water (unsweetened)
- Coffee (if preferred, without excessive added sugars)

Snacks:
- Raw vegetables (carrot sticks, cucumber slices)
- Hummus
- Greek yogurt (unsweetened)
- Cheese sticks (in moderation)
- Nut butter (unsweetened)

Frozen Foods:
- Frozen berries (for smoothies)
- Frozen vegetables (broccoli, spinach)
- Frozen fish filets

Sweeteners:
- Stevia or monk fruit sweetener (if needed)
- Honey or maple syrup (in moderation)

Miscellaneous:
- Herbs and spices for flavoring (rosemary, thyme, cumin, etc.)
- Whole-grain crackers or rice cakes
- Low-sodium broth (vegetable or chicken)
- Canned tomatoes (no added sugar)

- Whole-grain tortillas

This sample grocery list provides a balance of macronutrients and incorporates a range of flavors. Adjust quantities based on personal preferences, dietary requirements, and individual health goals. Regularly reviewing and updating the grocery list ensures that it aligns with changing dietary needs and preferences.

Quick and healthy recipes

1. Grilled Chicken and Vegetable Skewers:

Ingredients:
- Skinless chicken breasts, cut into cubes
- Bell peppers (variety of colors), cut into chunks
- Cherry tomatoes
- Zucchini, sliced
- Olive oil
- Garlic powder, paprika, salt, and pepper (to taste)

Instructions:
1. Preheat the grill or grill pan.
2. In a bowl, toss chicken cubes and vegetables with olive oil and seasonings.
3. Thread chicken and vegetables onto skewers.
4. Grill for 10-12 minutes, turning occasionally, until the chicken is cooked through and vegetables are tender.

2. Quinoa and Black Bean Salad:

Ingredients:
- Cooked quinoa
- Black beans, rinsed and drained
- Cherry tomatoes, halved
- Cucumber, diced
- Red onion, finely chopped
- Fresh cilantro, chopped
- Lime juice, olive oil, cumin, salt, and pepper (to taste)

Instructions:
1. In a large bowl, combine quinoa, black beans, tomatoes, cucumber, and red onion.
2. In a small bowl, whisk together lime juice, olive oil, cumin, salt, and pepper.
3. Pour the dressing over the salad and toss to combine.
4. Garnish with fresh cilantro before serving.

3. Baked Salmon with Lemon and Dill:

Ingredients:
- Salmon filets
- Lemon slices
- Fresh dill, chopped
- Garlic powder, salt, and pepper (to taste)

Instructions:
1. Preheat the oven to 400°F (200°C).
2. Place salmon filets on a baking sheet lined with parchment paper.
3. Season salmon with garlic powder, salt, and pepper.
4. Top each filet with lemon slices and sprinkle with fresh dill.
5. Bake for 15-20 minutes or until the salmon flakes easily with a fork.

4. Stir-Fried Vegetable Tofu Bowl:

Ingredients:
- Extra-firm tofu, cubed
- Broccoli florets
- Carrots, julienned
- Snap peas
- Bell peppers (variety of colors), sliced
- Low-sodium soy sauce
- Sesame oil
- Garlic, minced
- Ginger, grated
- Brown rice (cooked)

Instructions:
1. In a wok or skillet, heat sesame oil over medium-high heat.
2. Add tofu cubes and stir-fry until golden brown. Remove tofu from the pan.
3. In the same pan, add a bit more sesame oil if needed and sauté garlic and ginger.
4. Add broccoli, carrots, snap peas, and bell peppers. Stir-fry until vegetables are tender-crisp.
5. Add cooked tofu back to the pan, along with low-sodium soy sauce. Toss to combine.
6. Serve over brown rice.

5. Greek Yogurt Parfait:

Ingredients:
- Greek yogurt (unsweetened)
- Mixed berries (strawberries, blueberries, raspberries)
- Almonds or walnuts, chopped
- Honey or stevia (optional for sweetness)

Instructions:
1. In a glass or bowl, layer Greek yogurt.
2. Add a layer of mixed berries.
3. Sprinkle chopped nuts on top.
4. Drizzle with honey or add a pinch of stevia for sweetness if desired.

6. Veggie Omelette:

Ingredients:
- Eggs
- Bell peppers (variety of colors), diced
- Spinach, chopped
- Cherry tomatoes, halved
- Feta cheese (optional)
- Olive oil
- Salt and pepper (to taste)

Instructions:
1. In a bowl, whisk eggs and season with salt and pepper.
2. Heat olive oil in a non-stick skillet over medium heat.
3. Add diced bell peppers, spinach, and cherry tomatoes to the skillet and sauté until vegetables are tender.
4. Pour the whisked eggs over the vegetables, allowing them to set for a moment.
5. Once the edges start to set, gently lift with a spatula to let the uncooked egg flow underneath.
6. When the omelet is mostly set, sprinkle it with feta cheese if desired, then fold it in half.
7. Cook until the eggs are fully cooked through.

7. Chickpea and Vegetable Stir-Fry:

Ingredients:
- Chickpeas (canned, drained and rinsed)
- Broccoli florets
- Snow peas
- Carrots, sliced
- Red bell pepper, sliced
- Low-sodium teriyaki sauce
- Garlic, minced
- Ginger, grated
- Brown rice (cooked)

Instructions:
1. In a wok or skillet, heat a small amount of oil over medium-high heat.
2. Add minced garlic and grated ginger, sauté for a minute.
3. Add broccoli, snow peas, carrots, and red bell pepper. Stir-fry until vegetables are crisp-tender.
4. Add chickpeas and low-sodium teriyaki sauce. Stir to combine.
5. Serve over cooked brown rice.

8. Turkey and Vegetable Lettuce Wraps:

Ingredients:
- Lean ground turkey
- Iceberg or romaine lettuce leaves
- Bell peppers (variety of colors), diced
- Carrots, julienned
- Water chestnuts, chopped
- Low-sodium soy sauce
- Garlic, minced
- Ginger, grated

Instructions:
1. In a skillet over medium heat, cook ground turkey until browned.
2. Add minced garlic and grated ginger to the skillet.

3. Add diced bell peppers, julienned carrots, and water chestnuts. Sauté until vegetables are tender.
4. Stir in low-sodium soy sauce and cook until heated through.
5. Spoon the turkey and vegetable mixture into lettuce leaves to create wraps.

9. Berry and Spinach Salad:
 Ingredients:
- Spinach leaves
- Mixed berries (strawberries, blueberries, raspberries)
- Goat cheese or feta cheese (optional)
- Walnuts, chopped
- Balsamic vinaigrette dressing (low-sugar)

Instructions:
1. In a large bowl, combine spinach leaves, mixed berries, and optional cheese.
2. Sprinkle chopped walnuts over the top.
3. Drizzle with balsamic vinaigrette dressing and toss to coat.

10. Sweet Potato and Black Bean Bowl:

Ingredients:
- Sweet potatoes, cubed
- Black beans (canned, drained and rinsed)
- Avocado, sliced
- Cherry tomatoes, halved
- Cilantro, chopped
- Lime juice
- Cumin, paprika, salt, and pepper (to taste)

Instructions:
1. Roast cubed sweet potatoes in the oven until tender.
2. In a bowl, combine roasted sweet potatoes, black beans, cherry tomatoes, and sliced avocado.
3. Sprinkle with chopped cilantro.
4. Drizzle with lime juice and season with cumin, paprika, salt, and pepper.

These recipes are not only quick to prepare but also incorporate a balance of macronutrients, fiber, and essential nutrients, making them suitable for individuals managing Type 2 diabetes. Adjust portion sizes based on individual needs and preferences.

Chapter 4: 7 Days Meal Plan

In this chapter, this book provides a comprehensive 7 days meal plan designed to support individuals managing Type 2 diabetes. This plan incorporates the principles of balanced nutrition, portion control, and a variety of nutrient-dense foods to help regulate blood sugar levels, maintain a healthy weight, and promote overall well-being. Before starting any new meal plan, it's essential to consult with a healthcare professional or a registered dietitian to ensure it aligns with individual health needs and preferences.

Day 1: Balanced Start

Breakfast:
- Greek Yogurt Parfait:
  - Greek yogurt (unsweetened)
  - Mixed berries (strawberries, blueberries, raspberries)
  - Almonds or walnuts, chopped
  - Drizzle of honey or stevia (optional)

Lunch:
- Quinoa and Black Bean Salad:**
  - Quinoa
  - Black beans, rinsed and drained
  - Cherry tomatoes, halved
  - Cucumber, diced
  - Red onion, finely chopped
  - Fresh cilantro, chopped
  - Lime juice, olive oil, cumin, salt, and pepper

Dinner:
- Grilled Chicken and Vegetable Skewers:**
  - Skinless chicken breasts, cubed
  - Bell peppers (variety of colors), chunks
  - Cherry tomatoes
  - Zucchini, sliced
  - Olive oil, garlic powder, paprika, salt, and pepper

Day 2: Flavorful Variety

Breakfast:
- Vegetable Omelet:
  - Eggs
  - Bell peppers, diced
  - Spinach, chopped
  - Cherry tomatoes, halved
  - Feta cheese (optional)
  - Olive oil, salt, and pepper

Lunch:
-Stir-Fried Vegetable Tofu Bowl
  - Extra-firm tofu, cubed
  - Broccoli florets
  - Carrots, julienned
  - Snap peas
  - Bell peppers (variety of colors), sliced
  - Low-sodium soy sauce, sesame oil, garlic, and ginger
  - Brown rice (cooked)

Dinner:
- Baked Salmon with Lemon and Dill:
  - Salmon filets
  - Lemon slices
  - Fresh dill, chopped
  - Garlic powder, salt, and pepper

Day 3: Simple and Satisfying

Breakfast:
- Oatmeal with Berries and Nuts:
  - Rolled oats
  - Mixed berries (strawberries, blueberries)
  - Almonds or walnuts, chopped
  - Cinnamon and a splash of almond milk

Lunch:
- Turkey and Vegetable Lettuce Wraps:
  - Lean ground turkey
  - Iceberg or romaine lettuce leaves
  - Bell peppers, diced
  - Carrots, julienned
  - Water chestnuts, chopped
  - Low-sodium soy sauce, garlic, and ginger

Dinner:
- Chickpea and Vegetable Stir-Fry:
  - Chickpeas, canned, drained, and rinsed
  - Broccoli florets
  - Snow peas
  - Carrots, sliced
  - Red bell pepper, sliced
  - Low-sodium teriyaki sauce, garlic, and ginger
  - Brown rice (cooked)

Day 4: Abundant Colors and Flavors

Breakfast:
- Smoothie Bowl:
  - Spinach leaves
  - Mixed berries (strawberries, blueberries, raspberries)
  - Greek yogurt (unsweetened)
  - Chia seeds and a drizzle of honey

Lunch:
- Sweet Potato and Black Bean Bowl:
  - Sweet potatoes, cubed and roasted
  - Black beans, canned, drained, and rinsed
  - Avocado, sliced
  - Cherry tomatoes, halved
  - Cilantro, chopped
  - Lime juice, cumin, paprika, salt, and pepper

Dinner:
- Vegetarian Chili:
  - Kidney beans, black beans, and pinto beans (canned, drained, and rinsed)
  - Tomatoes, diced
  - Onion, chopped
  - Bell peppers (variety of colors), chopped
  - Garlic, minced
  - Chili powder, cumin, paprika, and vegetable broth

Day 5: Nourishing Choices

Breakfast:
- Chia Seed Pudding:
  - Chia seeds
  - Almond milk (unsweetened)
  - Mixed berries (strawberries, blueberries)
  - Almonds or walnuts, chopped

Lunch:
- Mediterranean Chickpea Salad:
  - Chickpeas, canned, drained, and rinsed
  - Cucumber, diced
  - Cherry tomatoes, halved
  - Kalamata olives, sliced
  - Red onion, finely chopped
  - Feta cheese (optional)
  - Olive oil, lemon juice, oregano, salt, and pepper

Dinner:
- Grilled Shrimp and Vegetable Kabobs:
  - Shrimp, peeled and deveined
  - Zucchini, cherry tomatoes, bell peppers
  - Olive oil, garlic, lemon juice, salt, and pepper

Day 6: Wholesome Delights

Breakfast
- Whole Grain Pancakes with Berries:
  - Whole grain pancake mix
  - Mixed berries (strawberries, blueberries)
  - Maple syrup (in moderation)

Lunch:
- Caprese Salad with Grilled Chicken:
  - Grilled chicken breast
  - Tomatoes, sliced
  - Fresh mozzarella, sliced
  - Basil leaves
  - Balsamic glaze, olive oil, salt, and pepper

Dinner:
- Baked Cod with Roasted Vegetables
  - Cod filets
  - Broccoli, carrots, cauliflower (roasted)
  - Olive oil, garlic, lemon zest, salt, and pepper

Day 7: Comforting and Satisfying

Breakfast:
- Vegetable and Cheese Frittata:
  - Eggs
  - Spinach, bell peppers, onions (sautéed)
  - Feta or goat cheese (optional)
  - Olive oil, salt, and pepper

Lunch:
- Turkey and Vegetable Soup:
  - Lean ground turkey
  - Carrots, celery, onions, garlic (chopped)
  - Low-sodium chicken broth, thyme, oregano, salt, and pepper

Dinner:
- Stuffed Bell Peppers with Quinoa and Black Beans:

- Bell peppers
- Quinoa, black beans, corn, tomatoes (mixed)
- Cumin, chili powder, garlic powder, salt, and pepper

Tips For Portion Control

➢ Use Smaller Plates and Bowls:
Opt for smaller dishware to create the illusion of a fuller plate. This can help control portion sizes and prevent overeating.

➢ Measure Portions:
Use measuring cups, spoons, or a food scale to measure ingredients and ensure accurate portion sizes.

➢ Follow the Plate Method:
Divide your plate into sections: half for non-starchy vegetables, one-quarter for lean protein, and one-quarter for whole grains or starchy vegetables.

➢ Be Mindful of Liquid Calories:
Be aware of the calories in beverages, including sugary drinks and alcohol. Choose water, herbal tea, or other low-calorie options.

➢ Listen to Hunger and Fullness Cues:
Pay attention to your body's signals. Eat slowly and stop when you feel satisfied, not overly full.

➢ Pre-portion Snacks:
Divide snacks into smaller portions rather than eating directly from the bag. This helps prevent mindless eating.

➢ Include a Variety of Foods:
Enjoy a variety of nutrient-dense foods to ensure you get a range of essential nutrients without overdoing it on any one type of food.

➢ Use Visual Cues:
Visual cues can help estimate portion sizes. For example, a serving of meat should be about the size of a deck of cards.

➢ Plan and Prepare Meals:
Plan meals ahead of time and portion out servings before sitting down to eat. This can prevent overeating and make it easier to manage portions.

➤ Practice Portion Control at Restaurants:

When dining out, consider splitting entrees with a dining partner, ordering appetizers as a main course, or asking for a to-go box at the beginning of the meal to set aside a portion.

➤ Limit Highly Processed Foods:

Processed foods often come in larger, less controllable portions. Focus on whole, unprocessed foods for better portion control.

➤ Understand Serving Sizes:

Familiarize yourself with standard serving sizes, as listed on food labels. This can help you make informed choices about portion control.

➤ Keep a Food Diary:

Tracking what you eat in a food diary can help raise awareness of portion sizes and identify patterns of overeating.

Chapter 5: The Power of Physical Activity

Physical activity is an incredibly powerful tool for managing Type 2 diabetes, and yet it is often overlooked. The benefits of regular physical activity extend far beyond weight management, positively influencing various aspects of overall health. Incorporating physical activity into one's routine can significantly improve blood sugar control, enhance insulin sensitivity, and contribute to a healthier lifestyle. Here are some key points that highlight the power of physical activity in managing Type 2 diabetes:

1. Improved Insulin Sensitivity:
Exercise helps to increase the body's sensitivity to insulin, the hormone responsible for regulating blood sugar. This means that the body can use insulin more effectively, helping to control blood glucose levels.

2. Blood Sugar Regulation:
Physical activity helps to lower blood sugar levels by promoting the uptake of glucose by muscle cells. This effect continues even after the exercise session, contributing to more stable blood sugar levels throughout the day.

3. Weight Management:
Maintaining a healthy weight is essential for managing Type 2 diabetes. Exercise aids in weight loss or weight maintenance by burning calories and promoting the development of lean muscle mass.

4. Cardiovascular Health:
Individuals with Type 2 diabetes are at an increased risk of cardiovascular diseases. Regular physical activity improves cardiovascular health by reducing the risk factors associated with heart disease, such as high blood pressure and cholesterol levels.

5. Enhanced Mood and Mental Well-being:
Exercise stimulates the release of endorphins, the body's natural mood lifters. Engaging in physical activity has been linked to reduced stress, anxiety, and depression, contributing to overall mental well-being.

6. Increased Energy Levels:

Regular physical activity improves energy levels and reduces fatigue, making day-to-day activities more manageable. This increase in energy can positively impact daily life, work, and social interactions.

7. Better Sleep Quality:
A consistent exercise routine is associated with improved sleep quality. Quality sleep is essential for overall health and can positively influence blood sugar control.

8. Muscle Strength and Flexibility:
Strength training exercises, combined with aerobic activities, enhance muscle strength and flexibility. This is particularly beneficial for individuals with Type 2 diabetes, as improved muscle function aids in better glucose metabolism.

9. Long-term Health Benefits:
Engaging in regular physical activity is linked to long-term health benefits, including a reduced risk of complications related to Type 2 diabetes, such as nerve damage, kidney disease, and eye problems.

10. Individualized Approach:
It's essential to tailor the exercise routine to individual preferences, fitness levels, and health conditions. Consulting with healthcare professionals or fitness experts can help design a safe and effective exercise plan.

Exercise for Type 2 Diabetes: A Comprehensive Guide to Suitable Activities

Physical activity is a cornerstone in the management of Type 2 diabetes, offering a myriad of benefits that contribute to better glucose control, improved cardiovascular health, and overall well-being. When crafting an exercise routine for individuals with Type 2 diabetes, it's crucial to consider factors such as individual fitness levels, health conditions, and personal preferences. This guide explores various types of exercises suitable for individuals with Type 2 diabetes, emphasizing the importance of a well-rounded approach to physical activity.

1. Aerobic Exercises:

Aerobic exercises, also known as cardiovascular exercises, involve continuous and rhythmic activities that elevate the heart rate. These exercises are crucial for improving cardiovascular health, aiding in weight management, and enhancing insulin sensitivity.

Examples:
- Brisk Walking: An accessible and effective form of aerobic exercise. Start with a moderate pace and gradually increase intensity.

- Cycling: Whether outdoors or using a stationary bike, cycling is a low-impact exercise that provides cardiovascular benefits.

- Swimming: A gentle yet effective full-body workout. Swimming is easy on the joints and suitable for individuals with mobility limitations.

- Dancing: Engaging in dance classes or following dance routines at home adds a fun and social element to aerobic exercise.

Benefits:
- Improves cardiovascular health.
- Aids in weight management.
- Enhances insulin sensitivity.
- Boosts mood and reduces stress.

2. Strength Training:

Strength or resistance training involves working against resistance to build and tone muscles. This type of exercise is vital for individuals with Type 2 diabetes as it contributes to improved glucose metabolism and overall metabolic health.

Examples:

- Weight Lifting: Incorporating free weights or weight machines into a routine builds muscle strength.

- Bodyweight Exercises: Exercises like squats, lunges, and push-ups use the body's own weight for resistance.

- Resistance Bands:These versatile bands provide resistance and can be used for a variety of strength exercises.

Benefits:
- Increases muscle mass.
- Enhances insulin sensitivity.
- Aids in weight management.
- Improves overall metabolic health.

3. Flexibility and Stretching:

Flexibility exercises involve stretching and lengthening muscles, contributing to improved range of motion and preventing injury. These exercises are essential for maintaining joint health and flexibility.

Examples
- Yoga: Combining physical postures, breathing exercises, and meditation, yoga enhances flexibility and reduces stress.

- Pilates: Focuses on core strength, flexibility, and overall body awareness.

- Static Stretching: Holding stretches for a set duration helps improve flexibility.

Benefits:
- Improves flexibility and range of motion.

- Aids in joint health.
- Reduces the risk of injury.
- Enhances relaxation and stress reduction.

4. Balance and Stability Training:

Balance and stability exercises are crucial, especially for older individuals with Type 2 diabetes, as they help prevent falls and injuries. These exercises improve coordination and enhance proprioception.

Examples:
- Tai Chi: A low-impact exercise that combines slow, flowing movements with deep breathing.

- Single-leg Stands:Simple exercises like standing on one leg help improve balance.

- Bosu Ball Exercises: Using a half stability ball adds an element of instability, engaging core muscles.

Benefits:
- Reduces the risk of falls and injuries.
- Enhances coordination and proprioception.
- Strengthens core muscles.

5. Interval Training:

Interval training involves alternating between short bursts of intense activity and periods of rest or lower-intensity exercise. This method is effective for burning calories, improving cardiovascular fitness, and managing blood sugar levels.

Examples:
- High-Intensity Interval Training (HIIT):** Short bursts of intense exercise (e.g., sprinting) followed by brief periods of rest or lower-intensity exercise.

- Circuit Training: Moving through a series of exercises with minimal rest between each.

Benefits:
- Burns calories efficiently.
- Improves cardiovascular fitness.
- Enhances insulin sensitivity.
- Time-efficient workout option.

6. Adaptive and Modified Exercises:

For individuals with specific health considerations or mobility limitations, adaptive and modified exercises can be tailored to suit their needs. These exercises are designed to accommodate various fitness levels and health conditions.

Examples:
- Chair Exercises: Seated exercises provide a workout for individuals with limited mobility or balance issues.

- Water Aerobics:Buoyancy in water reduces impact on joints, making exercises more accessible.

- Gentle Yoga or Tai Chi: Modified versions of these activities cater to individuals with reduced mobility or flexibility.

Benefits:
- Provides accessible options for diverse fitness levels.
- Accommodates individuals with specific health concerns.
- Promotes inclusivity and participation.

Tips for Safe Exercise

1. Consult with Healthcare Professionals:
   - Before starting a new exercise program, consult with healthcare providers, especially if you have existing health conditions.

2. Start Gradually:
   - Begin with low-intensity exercises and gradually increase the intensity and duration as fitness levels improve.

3. Monitor Blood Sugar Levels:
   - Check blood sugar levels before and after exercise to understand how physical activity affects glucose levels.

4. Stay Hydrated:
   - Drink plenty of water before, during, and after exercise to stay hydrated.

5. Include Warm-up and Cool-down:
   - Warm-up before exercise and cool down afterward to prevent injury and aid recovery.

6. Listen to Your Body:
   - Pay attention to how your body responds to exercise. If something doesn't feel right, adjust or stop the activity.

7. Consistency is Key:
   - Aim for consistency rather than intensity.

7 days manageable exercise routine

Creating a manageable exercise routine for Type 2 diabetes involves a balanced combination of aerobic exercises, strength training, flexibility, and balance activities. It's important to start gradually, listen to your body, and make adjustments based on your individual fitness level. Always consult with healthcare professionals before beginning a new exercise routine, especially if you have existing health conditions. Here's a sample exercise routine for individuals with Type 2 diabetes:

Weekly Exercise Routine:

Day 1: Aerobic Exercise
- Activity: Brisk Walking
  - Duration: 20-30 minutes
  - Intensity: Moderate pace
- Tip: Incorporate walking into your daily routine, like walking to the store or taking the stairs.

Day 2: Strength Training
- Activity:Bodyweight Exercises
  - Exercises: Squats, Lunges, Push-ups
  - Sets/Reps:2 sets of 10-12 reps for each exercise
- Tip:Start with a manageable number of repetitions and gradually increase as you build strength.

Day 3: Rest or Light Activity
- Activity: Gentle Stretching or Yoga
  - Duration: 15-20 minutes
- Tip: Focus on stretching major muscle groups to enhance flexibility and reduce tension.

Day 4: Aerobic Exercise
- Activity: Cycling or Swimming
  - Duration: 20-30 minutes
  - Intensity: Moderate
- Tip: Choose an activity you enjoy to make it a sustainable part of your routine.

Day 5: Strength Training

- Activity: Resistance Band Exercises
  - Exercises: Bicep Curls, Leg Press, Shoulder Press
  - Sets/Reps: 2 sets of 10-12 reps for each exercise
- Tip: Use resistance bands for added challenge while maintaining joint-friendly movements.

Day 6: Flexibility and Balance
- Activity: Yoga or Tai Chi
  - Duration: 20-30 minutes
-Tip: Focus on poses that improve balance and flexibility, such as tree pose or warrior pose.

Day 7: Rest or Light Activity
- Activity: Gentle Walking or Restorative Yoga
  - Duration: 15-20 minutes
- Tip: Allow your body to recover and prepare for the upcoming week.

General Tips:

1. Warm-up and Cool Down:
   - Include a 5-10 minute warm-up before each session, such as light cardio or dynamic stretching. Cool down with static stretches to improve flexibility and reduce muscle soreness.

2. Stay Hydrated:
   - Drink water before, during, and after exercise to stay hydrated.

3. Listen to Your Body:
   - If you experience pain or discomfort, modify the exercise or stop. It's crucial to prioritize safety.

4. Monitor Blood Sugar Levels:
   - Check your blood sugar levels before and after exercise, especially if you're taking medications that can affect blood sugar.

5. Gradual Progression:

- Gradually increase the duration, intensity, or complexity of exercises as your fitness level improves. Avoid pushing yourself too hard too soon.

6. Mix It Up:
   - Keep your routine interesting by incorporating different activities. This not only challenges your body but also prevents boredom.

7. Seek Professional Guidance:
   - Consult with healthcare professionals, especially if you have specific health concerns. A fitness professional or physical therapist can provide tailored guidance.

8. Consistency is Key:
   - Aim for regular, consistent exercise rather than sporadic intense workouts. Consistency is crucial for long-term health benefits.

Chapter 6: Monitoring Blood Sugar Levels

Monitoring blood sugar levels is an essential part of managing Type 2 diabetes. Accurate and regular monitoring gives individuals the power to make informed decisions about their lifestyle, medication, and overall diabetes management. This chapter will provide you with the information you need to understand the importance of blood sugar monitoring, the methods used, and how it can help you maintain optimal health.

Why Monitor Blood Sugar Levels?

Monitoring blood sugar levels is like having a compass to guide you through diabetes management. Here are some of the reasons why it is so important:

1. Understanding Individual Patterns:

Blood sugar levels can change throughout the day due to various factors, such as meals, physical activity, stress, and medication. Monitoring helps you identify your own patterns and create tailored management strategies.

2. Adjusting Lifestyle Choices:

By observing how your blood sugar responds to different foods, activities, and stressors, you can make informed choices. This includes adjusting your meal plans, exercise routines, and stress management techniques.

3. Medication Management:

For those on diabetes medications, monitoring blood sugar levels helps assess the effectiveness of the prescribed regimen. It allows healthcare professionals to make necessary adjustments to medication dosages.

4. Preventing Complications:

Consistent monitoring helps detect blood sugar fluctuations early on. This proactive approach can help prevent complications associated with poorly controlled diabetes, such as neuropathy, retinopathy, and cardiovascular issues.

5. Empowering Self-Management:

Knowing how your daily choices affect your blood sugar levels gives you the power to take an active role in your diabetes management. It also fosters a sense of control and accountability.

5. Seek Professional Guidance:

Discuss blood sugar trends and patterns with healthcare providers. They can provide personalized recommendations based on the data.

6. Take Action:

Use blood sugar data to make informed decisions about lifestyle, medication, and overall diabetes management. If levels consistently fall outside the target range, consult with healthcare professionals for adjustments.

The Significance of Regular Monitoring in Managing Type 2 Diabetes

Regular monitoring of blood sugar levels is an essential part of managing Type 2 diabetes. It not only provides individuals with valuable insights into their condition, but also enables them to make informed decisions and take proactive measures for optimal health. The importance of regular monitoring goes beyond mere data collection; it gives individuals the power to take charge of their diabetes management journey. Here are some key reasons why regular monitoring is so important:

1. Recognizing Personal Patterns:

Regular monitoring allows individuals to recognize patterns and trends in their blood sugar levels. By tracking glucose fluctuations throughout the day, they can identify how different factors such as meals, physical activity, stress, and medication affect their blood sugar. This personalized understanding is essential for customizing lifestyle choices and interventions to individual needs.

2. Adapting Lifestyle Choices:

Blood sugar monitoring serves as a guide for making informed lifestyle choices. Observing how the body responds to different foods, exercise routines, and stressors gives individuals the ability to adjust their daily activities to better manage blood sugar levels. It provides a real-time feedback mechanism that encourages a proactive approach to diabetes self-management.

3. Optimizing Medication Management:

For those on diabetes medications, regular monitoring offers insights into the effectiveness of the prescribed regimen. It allows healthcare professionals to make necessary adjustments to medication dosages, ensuring that the treatment plan is tailored to individual needs. This iterative process of monitoring and adjusting contributes to a more precise and personalized approach to medication management.

4. Avoiding Complications:

Consistent blood sugar monitoring serves as an early warning system for potential complications associated with poorly controlled diabetes. Detecting and addressing abnormal blood sugar levels quickly helps prevent complications such as neuropathy, retinopathy, cardiovascular issues, and other diabetes-related health concerns. It puts individuals in a position to take proactive steps in protecting their long-term health.

5. Empowering Self-Management:

Regular monitoring fosters a sense of empowerment and responsibility in individuals with Type 2 diabetes. It shifts the focus from a passive approach to a more active and engaged role in managing one's health. Understanding how daily choices influence blood sugar levels instills a sense of control, promoting a positive mindset that is essential in dealing with the challenges of living with diabetes.

6. Facilitating Informed Decisions:

Blood sugar data serves as a compass for making informed decisions about daily activities. Whether it's choosing meals, planning exercise routines, or managing stress, individuals armed with accurate blood sugar information can make decisions that are in line with their health goals. This informed decision-making contributes to a comprehensive and individualized approach to diabetes management.

7. Creating a Comprehensive Health Picture:

Regular monitoring, when combined with other health metrics such as blood pressure, cholesterol levels, and A1c, contributes to a comprehensive picture of an individual's health. This integrated approach allows healthcare professionals to provide personalized recommendations for managing not only blood sugar but also overall well-being.

8. Encouraging Timely Intervention:

The real-time nature of blood sugar monitoring facilitates timely intervention. If individuals consistently observe readings outside the target range, they can seek timely guidance from healthcare professionals. This proactive approach minimizes the risk of prolonged periods of uncontrolled blood sugar, reducing the likelihood of complications.

Understanding Blood Glucose Meters: A Key Tool in Diabetes Management

Blood glucose meters are invaluable devices for individuals with diabetes, providing a convenient and accessible means to monitor blood sugar levels at home. These portable devices empower individuals to take an active role in their diabetes management by offering real-time insights into how various factors influence their blood glucose levels. This understanding is crucial for making informed decisions about lifestyle, medication, and overall health. In this discussion, we explore the components, functionality, and best practices associated with blood glucose meters.

Components of a Blood Glucose Meter:

1. Meter Device:

   The main handheld device that displays blood sugar readings. It typically includes a screen for displaying results, buttons for navigation, and sometimes a memory function to store previous readings.

2. Test Strips:

   Small, disposable strips that are inserted into the meter. These strips draw in a small blood sample, allowing the meter to analyze the glucose level. Each meter model usually requires specific test strips.

3. Lancet Device:

   A spring-loaded device used to prick the fingertip and obtain a small blood sample. Lancets are generally disposable, and their depth can often be adjusted based on individual comfort.

4. Control Solution (Optional)

   A liquid with a known glucose concentration used to check the accuracy of the meter and test strips. It helps ensure that the meter is providing accurate readings.

How Blood Glucose Meters Work:

1. Blood Sample Collection:

   A small blood sample is obtained by pricking the fingertip with the lancet device. Some meters allow for alternative sites, such as the forearm or palm.

2. Application to Test Strip:
   The blood drop is applied to the designated area on the test strip.

3. Chemical Reaction:
   The test strip contains chemicals that react with glucose in the blood. This reaction generates an electrical current.

4. Measurement by the Meter:
   The meter measures the electrical current and translates it into a numerical value, representing the blood glucose level. This value is displayed on the meter's screen.

Best Practices for Using Blood Glucose Meters:

1. Follow Manufacturer Instructions:
   Adhere to the specific instructions provided by the meter's manufacturer. This includes proper use of test strips, lancets, and the meter itself.

2. Calibrate the Meter:
   Some meters require calibration, especially when using a new box of test strips. Follow the calibration steps outlined in the user manual.

3. Ensure Cleanliness:
   Keep the meter and its components clean. Avoid any substance that could interfere with accurate readings, such as food, liquids, or dirt.

4. Use Fresh Lancets:
   Change lancets regularly to ensure a sharp, clean puncture. This minimizes discomfort and helps obtain an adequate blood sample.

5. Check Expiration Dates:
   Regularly check the expiration dates of test strips and control solutions (if used) to ensure accuracy.

6. Consistent Blood Sample Size:
   Consistency in blood sample size is crucial for accurate readings. Follow the instructions regarding the required blood volume.
7. Store Supplies Properly:

Proper storage of test strips and lancets is essential. Follow the recommended storage conditions to maintain their effectiveness.

8. Understand Error Messages:
Familiarize yourself with the meter's error messages and troubleshooting steps. Contact the manufacturer or healthcare provider if persistent issues arise.

9. Record and Analyze Readings:
Keep a log of your blood sugar readings and share them with healthcare providers during appointments. Analyzing trends over time provides valuable insights.

Choosing a Blood Glucose Meter:

1. Compatibility:
Ensure that the meter is compatible with the specific test strips it requires.

2. Ease of Use:
-Choose a meter with user-friendly features and clear instructions.

3. Data Storage:
- Consider meters with memory storage if you prefer to track and review past readings.

4. Accessibility:
Some meters offer features such as large buttons or audible instructions for individuals with visual or dexterity challenges.

5. Cost
Factor in the cost of both the meter and the test strips when selecting a device. Some meters may be covered by insurance.

6. Connectivity:
Certain meters can sync with smartphone apps or other devices, providing a more integrated approach to diabetes management.

Interpreting Blood Sugar Readings

Interpreting blood sugar readings is a crucial skill for individuals with diabetes. The numbers obtained from blood glucose meters provide valuable insights into how the body is responding to various factors such as food, physical activity, stress, and medication. Understanding these readings allows individuals to make informed decisions about their daily choices, contributing to effective diabetes management. In this discussion, we explore the key metrics, target ranges, and actionable steps associated with interpreting blood sugar readings.

Key Metrics in Blood Sugar Readings:

1. Fasting Blood Sugar (FBS):
   Definition:** FBS measures blood glucose levels after an overnight fast.
   Normal Range: 70-100 mg/dL
   Target for Individuals with Diabetes: 80-130 mg/dL

2. Postprandial Blood Sugar (PPBS):
   Definition: PPBS measures blood glucose levels two hours after a meal.
   Normal Range: Less than 140 mg/dL
   Target for Individuals with Diabetes: Less than 180 mg/dL

3. A1c Levels:
   Definition: A1c, or glycated hemoglobin, represents the average blood sugar level over the   past 2-3 months.
   Normal Range: Less than 5.7%
   Target for Individuals with Diabetes: Usually below 7%, but individual targets may vary.

Interpreting Blood Sugar Readings:

1. Within Target Range:
   Significance: Readings within the target range indicate that blood sugar levels are well-controlled.
   Action: Continue with the current management plan and lifestyle choices.

2. Above Target Range:

Significance: Elevated readings may suggest insufficient control of blood sugar.

Action: Consider reviewing dietary choices, increasing physical activity, or consulting with healthcare professionals for potential medication adjustments.

3. Consistently High Readings:

Significance: Persistent high readings may indicate the need for more aggressive management.

Action: Consult with healthcare professionals to evaluate the overall diabetes management plan, including medication adjustments and potential lifestyle modifications.

4. Below Target Range:

Significance: Low readings may suggest the need for adjustments in medication or lifestyle choices.

Action: Evaluate recent activities, including medication timing, meals, and exercise. If low readings persist, consult with healthcare professionals for guidance.

5. Variability in Readings:

Significance: Wide fluctuations in readings may indicate inconsistent blood sugar control.

Action: Analyze patterns and identify contributing factors. Adjust lifestyle choices and medication under healthcare professional guidance.

6. A1c Levels:

Significance: A1c provides a longer-term perspective on blood sugar control.

Action: Aim for regular A1c testing and discuss results with healthcare professionals. Adjust management strategies based on the trends observed.

Tips for Effective Interpretation:

1. Keep a Log:

Maintain a log of blood sugar readings along with details about meals, exercise, and medication. This log aids in identifying patterns over time.

2. Identify Trends:

Look for trends in blood sugar readings. Understanding how specific activities impact blood sugar helps in making targeted adjustments.

3. Regularly Review with Healthcare Professionals:

Share blood sugar log and A1c results with healthcare providers during regular check-ups. Collaborate on adjusting the diabetes management plan as needed.

4. Consider Time of Day:

Recognize that blood sugar levels may vary at different times of the day. This awareness helps in tailoring management strategies accordingly.

5. Account for Other Factors:

Consider external factors such as stress, illness, or changes in routine that can influence blood sugar levels. Adjustments may be needed during such periods.

Chapter 7: Medications and Treatment Options

Understanding the various medications and treatment options available is a critical aspect of managing Type 2 diabetes effectively. This chapter explores the diverse range of medications, insulin therapy, and lifestyle interventions designed to help individuals achieve optimal blood sugar control and overall well-being.

1. Oral Medications:

a. Metformin:
  Mechanism: Improves insulin sensitivity and reduces glucose production in the liver.
  Usage: Often the first-line medication for Type 2 diabetes.
   Considerations: Generally well-tolerated, but side effects may include gastrointestinal issues.

b. Sulfonylureas:
  Mechanism: Stimulate the pancreas to produce more insulin.
  Usage: Can be used alone or in combination with other medications.
  Considerations: Risk of hypoglycemia; effectiveness may diminish over time.

c. DPP-4 Inhibitors:
  Mechanism: Increases insulin release and reduces glucose production.
  Usage: Often prescribed as an add-on to other medications.
   Considerations: Generally well-tolerated; may be used in combination with other drug classes.

d. SGLT-2 Inhibitors:
   Mechanism: Reduce glucose reabsorption in the kidneys, leading to increased excretion of glucose in urine.
  Usage: Can be used alone or in combination with other medications.
   Considerations: May be associated with lower cardiovascular risk; monitor for genital infections and dehydration.

e. GLP-1 Receptor Agonists
   Mechanism: Increase insulin release, decrease glucagon production, and slow gastric emptying.
  Usage: Often prescribed for those needing additional blood sugar control.

Considerations: May lead to weight loss; injectable options are available.

2. Insulin Therapy:

a. Rapid-Acting Insulin:
   Usage: Administered just before or after meals to control postprandial glucose levels.
   Considerations: Mimics the body's natural insulin response.

b. Short-Acting (Regular) Insulin:
   Usage: Typically taken 30 minutes before meals to control glucose throughout the day.
   Considerations: Less commonly used due to the availability of rapid-acting insulin.

c. Intermediate-Acting Insulin:
   Usage: Provides a longer duration of action; often taken in conjunction with rapid-acting insulin.
   Considerations: Offers coverage between meals and overnight.

d. Long-Acting Insulin:
   Usage: Provides a consistent level of insulin throughout the day and night.
   Considerations: Administered once or twice daily, offering basal insulin coverage.

e. Premixed Insulin:
   Usage: Combines a rapid- or short-acting insulin with an intermediate-acting insulin.
   Considerations: Convenient for individuals with consistent mealtime patterns.

3. Lifestyle Interventions:

a. Dietary Management:
   Focus: Emphasis on a balanced diet, portion control, and carbohydrate monitoring.
   Considerations:** Collaboration with a registered dietitian can provide personalized guidance.

b. Physical Activity:
   Benefits: Improves insulin sensitivity, aids in weight management, and contributes to overall cardiovascular health.
   Considerations: Consistency is key; consult with healthcare professionals before starting a new exercise routine.

c. Weight Management:

Goals: Achieving and maintaining a healthy weight can positively impact blood sugar control.

Considerations: A multidisciplinary approach involving diet, exercise, and behavioral strategies.

4. Combination Therapies:

a. Dual Therapy:

Usage: Combining two oral medications with complementary mechanisms of action.
Considerations: Customized based on individual needs and responses.

b. Triple Therapy:

Usage: Incorporating three different classes of medications to address multiple aspects of glucose regulation.
Considerations:** Reserved for cases where dual therapy is insufficient.

Overview of common medications- Importance of adherence to prescribed treatment

Managing Type 2 diabetes often involves a combination of lifestyle modifications and medications to achieve optimal blood sugar control. Understanding the common medications prescribed for Type 2 diabetes and the crucial importance of adhering to the prescribed treatment plan is essential for effective disease management.

Common Medications for Type 2 Diabetes:

1. Metformin:
   Mechanism: Improves insulin sensitivity and reduces glucose production in the liver.
   Usage: Often the first-line medication for Type 2 diabetes.
   Considerations: Generally well-tolerated; side effects may include gastrointestinal issues.

2. Sulfonylureas:
   Mechanism: Stimulate the pancreas to produce more insulin.
   Usage: Can be used alone or in combination with other medications.
   Considerations: Risk of hypoglycemia; effectiveness may diminish over time.

3. DPP-4 Inhibitors:

   Mechanism: Increases insulin release and reduces glucose production.
   Usage: Often prescribed as an add-on to other medications.
   Considerations: Generally well-tolerated; may be used in combination with other drug classes.

4. SGLT-2 Inhibitors:
   Mechanism: Reduce glucose reabsorption in the kidneys, leading to increased excretion of glucose in urine.
   Usage: Can be used alone or in combination with other medications.
   Considerations: May be associated with lower cardiovascular risk; monitor for genital infections and dehydration.

5. GLP-1 Receptor Agonists:

Mechanism: Increase insulin release, decrease glucagon production, and slow gastric emptying.

Usage: Often prescribed for those needing additional blood sugar control.

Considerations: May lead to weight loss; injectable options are available.

6. Insulin Therapy:

Types: Rapid-acting, short-acting, intermediate-acting, long-acting, premixed.

Usage: Administered based on specific needs, often in combination with other medications.

Considerations: Requires careful monitoring and adjustments; may involve multiple daily injections.

Importance of Adherence to Prescribed Treatment

1. Blood Sugar Control:
   Significance: Adhering to the prescribed treatment plan helps maintain consistent blood sugar levels within the target range.

Benefit: Reduces the risk of complications associated with poorly controlled diabetes, such as cardiovascular issues, neuropathy, and retinopathy.

2. Prevention of Complications:
   Significance:** Consistent adherence to medications can prevent or delay the onset of diabetes-related complications.
   Benefit: Protects against long-term health issues and improves overall quality of life.

3. Improved Quality of Life:
   Significance: Effective blood sugar control contributes to an improved quality of life.
   Benefit: Individuals experience fewer symptoms related to fluctuating blood sugar levels, such as fatigue, excessive thirst, and frequent urination.

4. Reduced Healthcare Costs:
   Significance: Adherence to prescribed treatment may lead to fewer hospitalizations and emergency room visits.
   -Benefit: Reduces the economic burden associated with diabetes management.

5. Individualized Care:
   -Significance: Adherence allows healthcare professionals to tailor the treatment plan based on individual responses.

Benefit: Optimizes medication adjustments and lifestyle recommendations for personalized care.

6. Stable Mental Health:
   Significance: Consistent adherence to treatment can contribute to stable mental health.
   Benefit: Minimizes the stress and anxiety associated with managing an unpredictable condition.

7. Collaborative Disease Management:

Significance: Adherence fosters a collaborative relationship between individuals and healthcare providers.

Benefit: Enables open communication, timely adjustments to the treatment plan, and shared decision-making.

Challenges and Strategies for Adherence:

. Medication Side Effects:
  - Challenge: Some medications may have side effects that impact adherence.
  - Strategy: Regular communication with healthcare providers to address concerns and explore alternative medications if needed.

2. Complex Treatment Plans:
 - Challenge: Managing multiple medications and insulin regimens can be complex.
   -Strategy: Simplifying the treatment plan, providing clear instructions, and utilizing medication organizers.

3. Financial Constraints:
  - Challenge: Cost of medications may be a barrier to adherence.
  - Strategy: Exploring financial assistance programs, generic alternatives, or discussing concerns with healthcare providers.

4. Lifestyle Factors:
  - Challenge: Busy lifestyles or forgetfulness may impact adherence.
  - Strategy: Incorporating medications into daily routines, setting reminders, and involving family members or caregivers for support.

5. Cultural and Belief Influences:
  -Challenge: Cultural beliefs or personal beliefs may affect medication adherence.
  - Strategy: Engaging in open conversations with healthcare providers to address concerns and provide culturally sensitive care.

Possible Side Effects and Precautions

While medications play a crucial role in managing Type 2 diabetes, it's important to be aware of potential side effects and take necessary precautions. Understanding these aspects empowers individuals to make informed decisions, seek timely medical attention when needed, and work collaboratively with healthcare providers for optimal diabetes management.

Common Side Effects and Precautions:

1. Metformin:

- Common Side Effects:
    - Gastrointestinal issues (e.g., nausea, diarrhea).
- Precautions:
    - Take with meals to minimize gastrointestinal discomfort.
    - Stay hydrated, especially if experiencing diarrhea.

2. Sulfonylureas:

- Common Side Effects:
    - Hypoglycemia (low blood sugar), weight gain.
- Precautions:
    - Monitor blood sugar levels regularly.
    - Be aware of symptoms of hypoglycemia, such as dizziness and confusion.

3. DPP-4 Inhibitors:

- Common Side Effects:
    - Upper respiratory tract infections, joint pain.
- Precautions:
    - Report persistent joint pain to healthcare providers.
    - Monitor for signs of infections and seek medical attention if needed.

4. SGLT-2 Inhibitors:

- Common Side Effects:
    - Genital yeast infections, increased urination, dehydration.

- Precautions:
    - Maintain adequate fluid intake.
    - Practice good hygiene to prevent infections.

5. GLP-1 Receptor Agonists:

- Common Side Effects:
    - Nausea, vomiting, injection site reactions.
- Precautions:
    - Start with a lower dose and gradually increase to improve tolerance.
    - Rotate injection sites to minimize discomfort.

6. Insulin Therapy:

- Common Side Effects:
    - Hypoglycemia, weight gain.
- Precautions:
    - Consistently monitor blood sugar levels.
    - Adjust insulin doses based on lifestyle changes or as directed by healthcare providers.

General Precautions for Diabetes Medications:

1. Hypoglycemia:

- Precautions:
    - Educate family members and caregivers on recognizing and responding to hypoglycemia.
    - Always carry a source of fast-acting carbohydrates.

2. Renal Function Monitoring:

- Precautions:
    - Regularly assess kidney function, especially when taking medications like metformin.
    - Stay hydrated to support kidney health.

3. Cardiovascular Precautions:

- Precautions:

- Individuals with a history of cardiovascular issues should discuss medication choices with healthcare providers.
- Monitor blood pressure and cholesterol levels regularly.

4. Liver Function Monitoring:

- Precautions:
    - Regularly assess liver function, particularly with certain medications.
    - Report any signs of liver issues, such as jaundice or abdominal pain.

5. Pregnancy and Breastfeeding:

- Precautions:
    - Consult with healthcare providers before and during pregnancy.
    - Discuss the safety of medications during breastfeeding.

6. Allergic Reactions:

- Precautions:
    - Be aware of potential allergic reactions, such as rash or swelling.
    - Seek immediate medical attention for severe allergic symptoms.

7. Regular Monitoring:

- Precautions:
    - Engage in regular blood sugar monitoring as advised by healthcare providers.
    - Attend scheduled check-ups to assess overall health and medication effectiveness.

When to Seek Medical Attention:

It's essential to promptly seek medical attention if experiencing:

- Severe Hypoglycemia: Persistent confusion, seizures, or loss of consciousness.
- Allergic Reactions: Difficulty breathing, swelling of the face or throat, severe rash.
- Signs of Liver Or Kidney Issues: Jaundice, abdominal pain, changes in urine output.

Chapter 8: Coping with Emotional Challenges of Type 2 Diabetes

Living with Type 2 diabetes involves not only managing physical health but also navigating the emotional challenges that can arise. This chapter explores the emotional aspects of diabetes, offering insights, coping strategies, and support for individuals and their loved ones as they navigate the complex landscape of emotions associated with the condition.

Understanding Emotional Challenges:

1. Stigma and Self-Blame:

- Challenge: Individuals with diabetes may face societal stigma or self-blame, feeling as though they caused their condition.
- Insight: Diabetes is a complex condition influenced by genetics, lifestyle, and other factors. Blame and stigma are unproductive and can hinder emotional well-being.

2. Fear and Anxiety:

- Challenge: Fear of complications, anxiety about managing blood sugar levels, and concerns about the future can be overwhelming.
- Insight: Acknowledge these fears, but work towards understanding and managing them through education and support.

3. Depression:

- Challenge: Living with a chronic condition may contribute to feelings of sadness and depression.
- Insight: Recognizing the signs of depression and seeking professional support is crucial. Mental health is an integral part of overall well-being.

4. Social Isolation:

- Challenge: Managing diabetes may lead to social isolation due to dietary restrictions or the need for regular monitoring.
- Insight: Finding a balance between diabetes management and social engagement is essential. Open communication with friends and family can foster understanding and support.

5. Burnout:

- Challenge: The constant vigilance required in diabetes management can lead to burnout.
- Insight: It's okay to acknowledge and address burnout. Seeking support from healthcare providers, support groups, or mental health professionals is crucial.

Coping Strategies:

1. Education and Empowerment:

- Strategy: Learn about diabetes, its management, and the factors influencing blood sugar control. Knowledge empowers individuals to make informed decisions.

2. Open Communication:

- Strategy: Share feelings and concerns with healthcare providers, family, and friends. Open communication fosters understanding and support.

3. Build a Support System:

- Strategy: Connect with others who have diabetes through support groups or online communities. A supportive network can provide valuable insights and encouragement.

4. Set Realistic Goals:

- Strategy: Break down diabetes management goals into achievable steps. Celebrate small victories and progress.

5. Mindfulness and Stress Management:

- Strategy: Incorporate mindfulness practices, meditation, or stress-reducing activities into daily routines. Managing stress positively impacts emotional well-being.

6. Professional Support:

- Strategy: If emotional challenges become overwhelming, seek the support of mental health professionals who specialize in chronic illness and emotional well-being.

- Solution: Establishing a routine, utilizing medication reminders, and seeking support can enhance adherence.

3. Unhealthy Coping Mechanisms:

- Risk: Stress and anxiety may trigger unhealthy coping mechanisms, such as emotional eating or increased intake of sugary foods.
- Healthy Alternatives: Adopting healthier coping strategies, such as exercise, mindfulness, or engaging in hobbies, can positively influence diabetes management.

4. Impact on Lifestyle Choices:

- Effect: Chronic stress may lead to poor lifestyle choices, affecting diet, exercise, and sleep patterns.
- Intervention: Developing strategies to address stress empowers individuals to make healthier lifestyle choices.

Coping Strategies for Stress and Anxiety in Type 2 Diabetes

1. Mindfulness and Relaxation Techniques:

- Approach: Incorporate mindfulness practices, deep breathing exercises, or progressive muscle relaxation into daily routines.
- Benefit: These techniques promote relaxation, reduce stress hormones, and contribute to overall well-being.

2. Regular Physical Activity:

- Approach: Engage in regular exercise, such as walking, jogging, or yoga.
- Benefit: Physical activity not only improves blood sugar control but also acts as a natural stress reliever.

3. Balanced Diet:

- Approach: Adopt a balanced and nutritious diet, focusing on whole foods and appropriate portion sizes.
- Benefit: A well-balanced diet supports stable blood sugar levels and provides essential nutrients for overall health.

4. Establishing a Routine:

- Approach: Create a daily routine that includes dedicated time for diabetes management tasks.
- Benefit: A structured routine enhances consistency in medication adherence, meal planning, and physical activity.

5. Building a Support System:

- Approach: Share concerns and experiences with friends, family, or support groups.
- Benefit: A supportive network provides emotional assistance and practical advice, fostering a sense of community.

6. Therapeutic Interventions:

- Approach: Consider therapy or counseling to address underlying stressors and develop coping strategies.
- Benefit: Professional support offers a safe space for exploring emotions and acquiring tools for managing stress and anxiety.

7. Mind-Body Practices:

- Approach: Explore mind-body practices like meditation, tai chi, or guided imagery.
- Benefit: These practices promote relaxation, reduce stress, and contribute to an improved mental state.

Creating a Personalized Stress Management Plan

1. Self-Reflection:

- Step: Reflect on individual stressors related to diabetes management and general life.
- Action: Identify specific triggers and patterns that contribute to stress and anxiety.

2. Setting Realistic Goals:

- Step: Establish achievable goals for stress management.
- Action: Break down larger objectives into smaller, manageable steps to build a sense of accomplishment.

- Effect: Living with a chronic condition may contribute to mental health challenges, including depression.
- Intervention: Recognizing signs of mental health issues and seeking professional support are essential components of holistic diabetes care.

Coping Strategies for Emotional Well-Being:

1. Education and Empowerment:

- Empowerment: Learning about Type 2 diabetes, its management, and the factors influencing blood sugar control empowers individuals to take an active role in their care.

2. Open Communication:

- Connection: Sharing feelings and concerns with healthcare providers, family, and friends fosters understanding and builds a supportive network.

3. Support Systems:

- Community: Connecting with others who have diabetes through support groups or online communities provides a sense of shared experience and encouragement.

4. Mindfulness and Stress Management:

- Practice: Incorporating mindfulness practices, meditation, or stress-reducing activities into daily routines supports emotional well-being.

5. Professional Support:

- Guidance: Seeking support from mental health professionals who specialize in chronic illness and emotional well-being is crucial for addressing complex emotional challenges.

6. Self-Compassion:

- Mindset: Cultivating self-compassion and recognizing that managing diabetes is a continuous journey with ups and downs contributes to a positive mindset.

7. Goal Setting and Celebrating Progress:

- Achievement: Setting realistic goals and celebrating small victories contribute to a sense of accomplishment and positive reinforcement.

The Role of Healthcare Providers:

1. Holistic Approach:

- Understanding: Healthcare providers adopting a holistic approach to diabetes care recognize the importance of addressing emotional well-being alongside physical health.

2. Regular Check-Ins:

- Communication: Incorporating discussions about emotional health during regular check-ups promotes open communication and early intervention if needed.

3. Referral to Mental Health Professionals:

- Collaboration: Referring individuals to mental health professionals when emotional challenges arise ensures a comprehensive and collaborative approach to care.

Community and Advocacy:

1. Diabetes Awareness:

- Education: Advocating for diabetes awareness helps combat stigma and fosters a supportive community.

2. Empowering Others:

- Connection: Sharing personal stories of resilience and coping strategies empowers others facing similar emotional challenges.

Building a Support System: A Vital Pillar in Managing Type 2 Diabetes

Living with Type 2 diabetes is a journey that extends beyond individual efforts and self-management. Building a robust support system is a critical aspect of effectively navigating the challenges associated with this chronic condition. This exploration delves into the significance of a support network, strategies for building one, and the positive impact it can have on the emotional and practical aspects of managing Type 2 diabetes.

Understanding the Role of a Support System:

1. Emotional Support:

- Importance: Managing Type 2 diabetes can be emotionally taxing. A support system provides a safe space to share feelings, fears, and triumphs.
- Effect: Emotional support fosters a sense of understanding and empathy, reducing feelings of isolation.

2. Practical Assistance:

- Scenario: The day-to-day management of diabetes involves various tasks, from medication adherence to meal planning. Practical assistance from a support system can ease the burden.
- Benefit: Shared responsibilities contribute to a more manageable and less overwhelming diabetes management routine.

3. Motivation and Encouragement:

- Impact: Diabetes management requires commitment and persistence. Motivation and encouragement from a support system can be a powerful catalyst for maintaining a positive mindset.
- Result: Regular encouragement reinforces healthy habits and boosts overall well-being.

4. Information and Education:

- Resource: A well-informed support system can provide valuable insights and information about Type 2 diabetes.

- Advantage: Access to accurate information enhances collective understanding and enables more informed decision-making.

Strategies for Building a Support System:

1. Engage with Healthcare Providers:

- Initiative: Include healthcare providers as integral members of the support system.
- Role: Healthcare professionals offer guidance, monitor health progress, and provide educational resources.

2. Family and Friends:

- Open Communication: Foster open communication with family and friends about the challenges and needs associated with managing diabetes.
- Involvement: Involve loved ones in aspects of diabetes care, from meal preparation to exercise routines.

3. Join Diabetes Support Groups:

- Community: Connect with local or online diabetes support groups.
- Benefits: These groups offer a sense of community, shared experiences, and practical advice.

4. Utilize Technology:

- Apps and Platforms: Leverage technology for virtual support through apps, online forums, or social media groups.
- Accessibility: Technology facilitates real-time communication and resource-sharing with a diverse support community.

5. Educate Support System Members:

- Training: Ensure that members of the support system understand the basics of Type 2 diabetes.
- Empowerment: Educated supporters can actively contribute to better-informed decisions and actions.

6. Set Clear Expectations:

- Communication: Clearly communicate expectations and boundaries within the support system.
- Clarity: Establishing clear expectations helps prevent misunderstandings and ensures a cohesive and supportive environment.

7. Celebrate Achievements Together:

- Acknowledgment: Recognize and celebrate achievements, no matter how small.
- Positive Reinforcement: Positive reinforcement contributes to a sense of accomplishment and encourages continued efforts.

The Impact of a Support System on Diabetes Management:

1. Emotional Well-Being:

- Enhancement: A supportive network contributes to improved emotional well-being.
- Stress Reduction: Emotional support reduces stress, anxiety, and feelings of isolation, fostering a positive mindset.

2. Consistent Diabetes Management:

- Adherence: A support system can play a pivotal role in promoting consistent medication adherence and lifestyle modifications.
- Accountability: Shared responsibilities create a sense of accountability, ensuring that essential tasks are not overlooked.

3. Improved Health Outcomes:

- Collaboration: Collaboration within a support system positively influences health outcomes.
- Holistic Care: Collective efforts address various aspects of diabetes management, promoting a holistic approach.

4. Knowledge and Awareness:

- Resourcefulness: A well-informed support system enhances overall knowledge about Type 2 diabetes.
- Proactive Decision-Making: Access to accurate information empowers everyone involved to make proactive and informed decisions.

Maintaining and Nurturing the Support System:

1. Regular Communication:

- Check-Ins: Schedule regular check-ins with members of the support system.
- Open Dialogue: Keep communication lines open to address concerns, share updates, and discuss potential adjustments to the support plan.

2. Express Gratitude:

- Recognition: Express gratitude for the support provided by each member.
- Positive Reinforcement: Acknowledging contributions fosters a positive and appreciative atmosphere.

3. Adaptability:

- Flexibility: Be adaptable to changes in the diabetes management plan or individual circumstances.
- Problem-Solving: Collaborate on solutions and adjustments as needed.

4. Self-Care for Supporters:

- Recognition: Recognize that supporting someone with Type 2 diabetes can also be challenging.
- Encouragement: Encourage self-care practices among support system members to ensure a balanced and sustainable support dynamic.

Chapter 9: Preventing Complications in Type 2 Diabetes: A Comprehensive Guide

Living with Type 2 diabetes necessitates a proactive and vigilant approach to prevent complications that may arise from uncontrolled blood sugar levels. This chapter serves as a comprehensive guide to understanding potential complications, implementing preventive measures, and fostering a holistic approach to managing Type 2 diabetes for long-term well-being.

Understanding Potential Complications:

1. Cardiovascular Complications:

- Risk: Individuals with Type 2 diabetes have an increased risk of heart disease, including heart attacks and strokes.
- Prevention: Maintaining optimal blood pressure, cholesterol levels, and adopting a heart-healthy lifestyle are crucial preventive measures.

2. Neuropathy:

- Risk: Elevated blood sugar levels can damage nerves, leading to neuropathy, which may manifest as pain, tingling, or numbness, particularly in the extremities.
- Prevention: Strict blood sugar control, regular foot care, and lifestyle modifications arc kcy prcventive strategies.

3. Nephropathy:

- Risk: Diabetes can affect the kidneys, leading to nephropathy, a condition that may progress to kidney failure.
- Prevention: Blood sugar control, blood pressure management, and regular monitoring of kidney function are essential preventive measures.

4. Retinopathy:

- Risk: Diabetes can cause damage to the blood vessels in the eyes, leading to retinopathy and potential vision impairment.
- Prevention: Regular eye exams, blood sugar control, and blood pressure management contribute to preventing retinopathy.

5. Foot Complications:

- Risk: Diabetes-related nerve damage and poor circulation can lead to foot complications, including infections and ulcers.
- Prevention: Regular foot care, proper footwear, and early intervention for any foot issues are crucial preventive measures.

6. Infections and Wound Healing:

- Risk: Diabetes can weaken the immune system, making individuals more susceptible to infections and impairing wound healing.
- Prevention: Good hygiene practices, timely wound care, and proactive infection management are essential preventive strategies.

Holistic Approaches to Preventing Complications:

1. Blood Sugar Control:

- Optimal Levels: Maintaining blood sugar levels within the target range is the cornerstone of preventing complications.
- Regular Monitoring: Consistent monitoring and adjustments to medication or lifestyle ensure optimal control.

2. Blood Pressure Management:

- Target Range: Keeping blood pressure within the recommended range is vital for preventing cardiovascular and kidney complications.
- Lifestyle Changes: Adopting a low-sodium diet, regular exercise, and medication adherence contribute to blood pressure control.

3. Cholesterol Management:

- Healthy Levels: Maintaining healthy cholesterol levels is crucial for cardiovascular health.
- Diet and Medication: A heart-healthy diet and, if necessary, cholesterol-lowering medications play a role in prevention.

4. Healthy Lifestyle Choices:

- Nutrition: Adopting a balanced and nutritious diet, emphasizing whole foods and limiting processed sugars and saturated fats, is essential.
- Regular Exercise: Engaging in regular physical activity promotes overall well-being and helps control blood sugar levels.

5. Regular Medical Check-Ups:

- Comprehensive Assessments: Regular check-ups with healthcare providers include monitoring blood sugar, blood pressure, cholesterol, and assessing overall health.
- Early Detection: Early detection of potential issues allows for timely intervention and preventive measures.

6. Medication Adherence:

- Consistency: Adhering to prescribed medications as directed by healthcare providers is crucial for managing blood sugar levels and preventing complications.
- Communication: Open communication with healthcare providers about medication concerns or side effects is essential.

7. Quit Smoking and Limit Alcohol Intake:

- Impact on Complications: Smoking and excessive alcohol intake can exacerbate diabetes-related complications.
- Cessation Programs: Participating in smoking cessation programs and limiting alcohol intake contribute to overall health.

Empowering Individuals for Complication Prevention:

1. Education and Awareness:

- Informed Decision-Making: Providing comprehensive information empowers individuals to make informed decisions about their health.
- Understanding Risks: Awareness of the risks associated with Type 2 diabetes fosters a proactive approach to prevention.

2. Individualized Care Plans:

- Tailored Approaches: Healthcare providers should collaborate with individuals to create personalized care plans.

- Goals and Targets: Establishing specific goals and targets ensures a focused and achievable approach to prevention.

3. Psychosocial Support:

- Emotional Well-Being: Addressing psychosocial factors, such as stress and mental health, contributes to overall well-being and aids in complication prevention.
- Support Systems: A supportive network can play a crucial role in managing the emotional aspects of diabetes and maintaining focus on preventive measures.

4. Periodic Assessments and Adjustments:

- Regular Review: Periodic assessments of health parameters and adjustment of care plans based on changing needs are essential.
- Adaptability: Being adaptable and making necessary adjustments contribute to ongoing preventive efforts.

The Importance of Routine Check-Ups in Managing Type 2 Diabetes: Safeguarding Your Health

Routine check-ups play a pivotal role in the comprehensive management of Type 2 diabetes, serving as a proactive strategy to monitor and safeguard an individual's health. This exploration delves into the significance of regular medical assessments, the components of routine check-ups, and the positive impact they have on overall well-being for those navigating the complexities of Type 2 diabetes.

1. Early Detection of Complications:

- Key Benefit: Routine check-ups allow healthcare providers to detect potential complications associated with Type 2 diabetes at an early stage.
- Preventive Measures: Early identification enables timely intervention, preventive measures, and adjustments to the treatment plan to mitigate the impact of complications.

2. Monitoring Blood Sugar Levels:

- Crucial Aspect: Regular assessments include monitoring blood sugar levels, a fundamental aspect of diabetes management.
- Optimizing Control: Continuous monitoring provides insights into the effectiveness of the current treatment plan, facilitating adjustments for optimal blood sugar control.

3. Blood Pressure and Cholesterol Management:

- Cardiovascular Health: Routine check-ups include monitoring blood pressure and cholesterol levels, essential components of cardiovascular health.
- Preventive Strategies: These assessments guide healthcare providers in prescribing appropriate interventions and preventive strategies to reduce the risk of cardiovascular complications.

4. Kidney Function Monitoring:

- Nephropathy Prevention: Regular assessments include monitoring kidney function, crucial for preventing nephropathy associated with diabetes.
- Early Intervention: Identifying any signs of kidney impairment allows for early intervention to preserve kidney health.

5. Foot Examinations:

- Preventing Complications: Routine check-ups often involve foot examinations to detect early signs of neuropathy or circulation issues.
- Foot Care Education: Healthcare providers can offer guidance on proper foot care, reducing the risk of complications such as infections and ulcers.

6. Eye Exams:

- Retinopathy Detection: Regular eye exams are essential for detecting signs of retinopathy, a diabetes-related complication affecting the eyes.
- Preserving Vision: Early detection allows for timely interventions to preserve vision and manage any emerging eye-related issues.

7. Medication Management:

- Evaluating Effectiveness: Routine check-ups provide an opportunity to assess the effectiveness of prescribed medications.
- Adaptations if Needed: Healthcare providers can make adjustments to medication dosages or types based on an individual's response and changing health needs.

8. Behavioral and Lifestyle Assessment:

- Holistic Approach: Routine check-ups involve discussions about behavioral and lifestyle factors influencing diabetes management.
- Behavioral Counseling: Healthcare providers may offer behavioral counseling to address challenges, promote positive lifestyle changes, and enhance overall well-being.

9. Psychosocial Support:

- Addressing Mental Health: Routine check-ups create a platform for addressing psychosocial aspects, including stress and mental health concerns.
- Connecting to Resources: Healthcare providers can connect individuals with appropriate resources, support groups, or mental health professionals when needed.

10. Educational Opportunities:

- Empowering Individuals: Routine check-ups offer educational opportunities to empower individuals with information about Type 2 diabetes.

- Promoting Self-Care: Education encourages proactive self-care, fostering a sense of autonomy in managing the condition.

11. Building a Long-Term Relationship:

- Trust and Communication: Regular check-ups contribute to the development of a long-term relationship between individuals and healthcare providers.
- Effective Communication: Establishing trust and effective communication ensures that individuals feel comfortable discussing their concerns and collaborating on their care plan.

Recognizing Warning Signs in Type 2 Diabetes: A Vital Key to Timely Intervention

Understanding and recognizing warning signs is crucial for individuals managing Type 2 diabetes. Early detection of signs and symptoms allows for timely intervention, preventing the escalation of issues and promoting effective management. This exploration delves into common warning signs associated with Type 2 diabetes, the importance of vigilance, and strategies for prompt action to safeguard health.

1. Changes in Blood Sugar Levels:

- Symptoms: Frequent thirst, increased urination, and unexplained weight changes may indicate fluctuations in blood sugar levels.
- Action: Regular monitoring of blood sugar levels and prompt adjustments to medication or lifestyle can help maintain optimal control.

2. Fatigue and Weakness:

- Symptoms: Persistent fatigue and weakness could be indicative of uncontrolled diabetes or potential complications.
- Action: Seeking medical attention for a comprehensive assessment and adjustments to the treatment plan if necessary.

3. Frequent Infections:

- Symptoms: Individuals with diabetes may experience more frequent infections, such as urinary tract infections or skin infections.
- Action: Timely medical intervention to address the infection and review of diabetes management for potential adjustments.

4. Blurred Vision:

- Symptoms: Blurred or fluctuating vision may signal changes in blood sugar levels affecting the eyes.
- Action: Scheduling an eye exam promptly to detect and manage potential complications like retinopathy.

5. Numbness or Tingling:

- Symptoms: Numbness or tingling in the extremities may indicate neuropathy, a diabetes-related nerve condition.
- Action: Seeking medical evaluation for proper diagnosis and implementing preventive measures.

6. Unexplained Weight Loss:

- Symptoms: Unintended weight loss without changes in diet or physical activity may be a warning sign.
- Action: Consulting with healthcare providers to investigate and address potential underlying issues.

7. Increased Hunger:

- Symptoms: Experiencing persistent hunger, especially shortly after eating, may signal imbalances in blood sugar levels.
- Action: Adjusting meal plans and discussing symptoms with healthcare providers for potential treatment modifications.

8. Slow Wound Healing:

- Symptoms: Slow healing of cuts or wounds may indicate impaired circulation or compromised immune function.
- Action: Seeking medical attention to address the wound promptly and evaluating overall diabetes management.

9. Increased Thirst and Dry Mouth:

- Symptoms: Excessive thirst and a dry mouth may result from elevated blood sugar levels.
- Action: Hydration and monitoring blood sugar levels, with adjustments as needed, can help alleviate symptoms.

10. Changes in Mood or Mental Function:

- Symptoms: Mood swings, irritability, or difficulty concentrating may be linked to fluctuations in blood sugar levels affecting mental function.
- Action: Seeking medical advice for evaluation and potential adjustments to diabetes management.

11. Changes in Skin Health:

- Symptoms: Dry skin, dark patches, or skin infections may indicate complications related to diabetes.
- Action: Regular skin checks and prompt medical attention for any concerning changes.

12. Increased Urination at Night:

- Symptoms: Frequent trips to the bathroom at night may be a sign of uncontrolled diabetes.
- Action: Adjusting fluid intake and discussing symptoms with healthcare providers for appropriate interventions.

Importance of Vigilance and Timely Intervention:

1. Preventing Complications:

- Rationale: Recognizing warning signs early can prevent the development or escalation of diabetes-related complications.
- Action: Timely medical intervention and adjustments to the diabetes management plan contribute to overall well-being.

2. Optimizing Blood Sugar Control:

- Benefit: Prompt action based on warning signs allows for optimization of blood sugar control.
- Empowerment: Individuals can actively participate in their diabetes management by responding proactively to changes in symptoms.

3. Enhancing Quality of Life:

- Outcome: Early recognition and intervention contribute to maintaining a higher quality of life for individuals with Type 2 diabetes.
- Holistic Approach: Addressing warning signs comprehensively promotes physical and emotional well-being.

4. Preventive Measures for Complications:

- Strategy: Recognizing warning signs enables the implementation of preventive measures to reduce the risk of complications.
- Holistic Care: A proactive approach includes lifestyle adjustments, medication management, and regular monitoring.

Strategies for Prompt Action:

1. Regular Monitoring:

- Empowerment: Individuals should engage in regular self-monitoring of blood sugar levels, especially when noticing changes in symptoms.
- Communication: Communicating findings with healthcare providers allows for informed decision-making.

2. Open Communication with Healthcare Providers:

- Collaboration: Establishing open communication with healthcare providers is crucial for sharing concerns and receiving timely guidance.
- Consultation: Seeking professional advice promptly contributes to effective management.

3. Adherence to Treatment Plans:

- Consistency: Adhering to prescribed treatment plans, including medications and lifestyle modifications, is essential.
- Regular Check-Ups: Routine check-ups facilitate ongoing assessments and adjustments to the treatment plan.

4. Education and Empowerment:

- Knowledge: Empowering individuals with knowledge about warning signs enhances their ability to recognize changes.
- Self-Advocacy: Education encourages individuals to advocate for their health and seek timely medical attention.

5. Holistic Lifestyle Management:

- Balanced Approach: Adopting a holistic approach to lifestyle management, including nutrition, exercise, and stress reduction, supports overall health.

- **Wellness Focus:** Prioritizing overall wellness contributes to better diabetes management and symptom recognition.

Strategies for Preventing Long-Term Complications in Type 2 Diabetes: A Comprehensive Guide

Preventing long-term complications in Type 2 diabetes requires a proactive and holistic approach to overall health management. This chapter explores essential strategies aimed at reducing the risk of complications, promoting optimal well-being, and empowering individuals to take charge of their diabetes journey for long-term health.

1. Blood Sugar Control:

- Target Range: Maintaining blood sugar levels within the target range is fundamental for preventing complications.
- Regular Monitoring: Consistent monitoring and adjustments to medication or lifestyle ensure optimal control.

2. Blood Pressure and Cholesterol Management:

- Cardiovascular Health: Controlling blood pressure and managing cholesterol levels are crucial for preventing cardiovascular complications.
- Lifestyle Modifications: Adopting a heart-healthy diet, regular exercise, and medication adherence contribute to cardiovascular well-being.

3. Regular Medical Check-Ups:

- Comprehensive Assessments: Regular check-ups with healthcare providers include monitoring blood sugar, blood pressure, cholesterol, and assessing overall health.
- Early Detection: Early detection of potential issues allows for timely intervention and preventive measures.

4. Lifestyle Modifications:

- Nutritious Diet: Adopting a balanced and nutritious diet, emphasizing whole foods and limiting processed sugars and saturated fats, is essential.
- Regular Exercise: Engaging in regular physical activity promotes overall well-being and helps control blood sugar levels.

5. Medication Adherence:

- Consistency: Adhering to prescribed medications as directed by healthcare providers is crucial for managing blood sugar levels and preventing complications.

- Communication: Open communication with healthcare providers about medication concerns or side effects is essential.

6. Quit Smoking and Limit Alcohol Intake:

- Impact on Complications: Smoking and excessive alcohol intake can exacerbate diabetes-related complications.
- Cessation Programs: Participating in smoking cessation programs and limiting alcohol intake contribute to overall health.

7. Weight Management:

- Healthy Weight: Maintaining a healthy weight reduces the risk of complications associated with obesity.
- Nutrition and Exercise: Combining a balanced diet with regular exercise supports weight management and overall health.

8. Foot Care:

- Regular Inspections: Regularly inspecting and caring for the feet helps prevent complications related to neuropathy and circulation issues.
- Proper Footwear: Wearing comfortable and supportive footwear contributes to foot health.

9. Eye Care:

- Regular Eye Exams: Routine eye exams detect early signs of retinopathy and other diabetes-related eye issues.
- Protection from UV Rays: Wearing sunglasses to protect the eyes from UV rays supports eye health.

10. Stress Management:

- Relaxation Techniques: Incorporating stress-reducing activities such as meditation, yoga, or deep breathing supports overall well-being.
- Balancing Priorities: Managing stress contributes to better mental and physical health.

11. Sleep Hygiene:

- Quality Sleep: Prioritizing good sleep hygiene ensures adequate rest, which is essential for overall health.
- Routine Sleep Schedule: Maintaining a consistent sleep schedule supports optimal well-being.

12. Regular Dental Care:

- Oral Health: Regular dental check-ups and proper oral care contribute to overall health and prevent complications related to gum disease.
- Hygiene Practices: Daily brushing and flossing help maintain oral hygiene.

13. Psychosocial Support:

- Mental Health Awareness: Addressing psychosocial factors, such as stress and mental health, is crucial for overall well-being.
- Support Systems: A supportive network can play a crucial role in managing the emotional aspects of diabetes and maintaining focus on preventive measures.

14. Regular Vaccinations:

- Preventive Measures: Staying up-to-date with vaccinations, including influenza and pneumonia vaccines, supports overall health.
- Consultation with Healthcare Providers: Discussing vaccination recommendations with healthcare providers ensures comprehensive preventive care.

15. Education and Empowerment:

- Informed Decision-Making: Providing comprehensive information empowers individuals to make informed decisions about their health.
- Lifelong Learning: Ongoing education encourages individuals to stay informed about the latest advancements in diabetes management and preventive strategies.

Chapter 10: Celebrating Success and Setting Future Goals in the Journey of Type 2 Diabetes Management

The journey of managing Type 2 diabetes is marked by milestones, challenges, and continuous growth. This chapter emphasizes the importance of celebrating successes, acknowledging progress, and setting future goals as integral components of a positive and empowering approach to diabetes management. By fostering a mindset of achievement and resilience, individuals can navigate their diabetes journey with confidence and purpose.

Celebrating Successes:

1. Recognition of Achievements:

- Importance: Taking a moment to recognize and celebrate achievements, whether big or small, is crucial for maintaining motivation and a positive mindset.
- Positive Reinforcement: Celebrating success provides positive reinforcement, encouraging individuals to stay committed to their diabetes management plan.

2. Improved Blood Sugar Control:

- Success Indicator: Achieving and maintaining optimal blood sugar levels is a significant success in diabetes management.
- Celebration: Recognizing improvements in HbA1c levels and consistent blood sugar control calls for celebration and acknowledgment of the hard work put into achieving this milestone.

3. Lifestyle Modifications:

- Success Stories: Successfully incorporating and sustaining lifestyle modifications, such as a balanced diet and regular exercise, are accomplishments worth celebrating.
- Healthy Habits: Commending the establishment of healthy habits reinforces the importance of these positive changes for long-term well-being.

4. Weight Management:

- Achievement: Attaining and maintaining a healthy weight is an accomplishment that contributes to overall health.
- Self-Reflection: Celebrating weight management success encourages self-reflection on the efforts made and the impact on diabetes management.

5. Consistent Medication Adherence:

- Adherence: Consistently adhering to prescribed medications is a significant success in maintaining blood sugar control.
- Acknowledgment: Acknowledging the commitment to medication adherence reinforces the importance of this aspect of diabetes care.

6. Routine Check-Up Milestones:

- Regular Assessments: Reaching milestones in routine check-ups, with positive feedback from healthcare providers, is a cause for celebration.
- Health Progress: Recognition of health progress during check-ups serves as a motivational boost for continued dedication to diabetes management.

Setting Future Goals:

1. Holistic Well-Being:

- Goal Setting: Setting future goals for holistic well-being encompasses physical, mental, and emotional health.
- Balanced Lifestyle: Goals may include maintaining a balanced lifestyle, managing stress, and fostering emotional resilience.

2. Advanced Blood Sugar Control:

- Progressive Goals: Continuously improving blood sugar control can be a progressive goal for individuals with Type 2 diabetes.
- Collaboration with Healthcare Providers: Collaborating with healthcare providers to establish realistic targets and strategies for ongoing improvement.

3. Lifelong Learning:

- Educational Goals: Setting goals for ongoing education about Type 2 diabetes and its management fosters empowerment.
- Information Gathering: Embracing a mindset of lifelong learning ensures individuals stay informed about the latest advancements in diabetes care.

4. Physical Activity Milestones:

- Diverse Goals: Establishing and achieving milestones in physical activity, whether it's increasing daily steps or exploring new forms of exercise, can be future goals.
- Adaptability: Goals should be adaptable to individual preferences and physical capabilities.

5. Nutritional Advancements:

- Continuous Improvement: Continually refining and advancing nutritional choices is a valuable goal for long-term health.
- Exploration: Exploring new recipes, incorporating diverse food groups, and finding joy in nourishing the body contribute to nutritional well-being.

6. Emotional Resilience:

- Mindfulness Goals: Incorporating mindfulness practices and stress management techniques into daily life can be a future goal.
- Coping Strategies: Setting goals for developing effective coping strategies enhances emotional resilience in the face of diabetes-related challenges.

7. Community Engagement:

- Social Connection: Setting goals for increased community engagement, whether through support groups or online forums, promotes a sense of belonging.
- Shared Experiences: Connecting with others who share similar experiences provides valuable support and encouragement.

8. Advocacy and Outreach:

- Empowerment Goals: Advocating for diabetes awareness and becoming an outreach advocate in the community can be a future goal.
- Impact: Sharing personal experiences and insights contributes to a broader understanding of Type 2 diabetes and reduces stigma.

The Cycle of Celebration and Goal Setting:

1. Cyclic Process:

- Continuous Improvement: The cycle of celebrating successes and setting future goals is a continuous and cyclic process.
- Feedback Loop: Each success becomes a feedback loop for motivation and inspiration to pursue new goals.

2. Adaptable Approach:

- Flexibility: The approach to celebrating successes and setting future goals should be adaptable to individual circumstances.
- Reassessment: Periodically reassessing goals ensures they align with evolving health needs and aspirations.

3. The Support System Involvement:

1. Family and Friends:

- Celebrating Together: Involving family and friends in the celebration of successes creates a supportive environment.
- Shared Goals: Engaging loved ones in the goal-setting process ensures a network of encouragement.

2. Healthcare Providers:

- Collaborative Planning: Collaborating with healthcare providers in both celebration and goal setting ensures a well-rounded approach.
- Professional Guidance: Regular consultations provide professional guidance for realistic goal setting and health assessment.

3. Support Groups:

- Shared Experiences: Being part of support groups or online communities allows individuals to share successes and gain insights.
- Collective Goal Setting: Setting collective goals within a supportive community fosters a sense of unity and shared accomplishment.

Mindset Shift and Reflection:

1. Mindset Transformation:

- Positive Outlook: Celebrating successes and setting future goals contribute to a positive mindset.
- Transformative Approach: Shifting from a focus on challenges to celebrating achievements cultivates resilience and determination.

2. Reflective Practices:

- Self-Reflection: Regular self-reflection on achievements and goals provides insights into personal growth.
- Adjustments: The ability to adjust goals based on self-reflection ensures they remain aligned with evolving priorities.

Creating Milestones and Rewards:

1. Milestone Recognition:

- Defining Milestones: Establishing specific milestones helps track progress and achievements.
- Recognition Rituals: Creating rituals for acknowledging milestones reinforces the significance of accomplishments.

2. Personalized Rewards:

- Customized Incentives: Setting up personalized rewards for reaching goals adds a motivational element.
- Healthy Rewards: Choosing rewards that align with overall health, such as a wellness retreat or a new fitness accessory, promotes a holistic approach.

Reflecting on the Past 30 Days: A Journey of Self-Discovery in Type 2 Diabetes Management

As we conclude the past 30 days, it's a valuable moment to pause, reflect, and appreciate the journey embarked upon in managing Type 2 diabetes. This chapter encourages a thoughtful examination of achievements, challenges, and personal growth over the past month. Through reflection, individuals can gain insights, celebrate successes, and pave the way for continued progress in their diabetes management.

Celebrating Achievements:

1. Blood Sugar Control:

- Monitoring Success: Reflecting on the past 30 days allows for an assessment of blood sugar control achievements.
- Consistent Efforts: Celebrating moments of optimal blood sugar levels and the consistency in monitoring efforts is a cause for acknowledgment.

2. Lifestyle Modifications:

- Dietary Triumphs: Reviewing dietary changes and healthier eating habits provides an opportunity for celebration.
- Exercise Milestones: Recognizing achievements in incorporating regular physical activity contributes to a sense of accomplishment.

3. Medication Adherence:

- Consistency Acknowledgment: Reflecting on adherence to prescribed medications offers a chance to acknowledge consistent efforts.
- Communication Success: Celebrating open communication with healthcare providers regarding medication experiences fosters a positive approach.

4. Routine Check-Ups:

- Feedback Reception: Considering feedback from routine check-ups and medical assessments allows for celebration.
- Progress Recognition: Acknowledging health progress and positive feedback from healthcare providers adds to the sense of achievement.

Navigating Challenges:

1. Learning Opportunities:

- Identification of Challenges: Reflecting on challenges encountered provides insight into areas that may require additional attention.
- Learning from Setbacks: Viewing challenges as learning opportunities sets the stage for future growth and adaptation.

2. Emotional Resilience:

- Mindset Reflection: Assessing emotional well-being and stress management highlights the importance of emotional resilience.
- Coping Strategies: Identifying effective coping strategies and areas for improvement contributes to ongoing mental health.

3. Adjusting Goals:

- Flexibility Acknowledgment: Recognizing the need for adjustments in goals showcases flexibility in the diabetes management journey.
- Adaptability: Embracing adaptability ensures that goals remain realistic and achievable in the face of changing circumstances.

Personal Growth and Insights:

1. Self-Discovery:

- Understanding Habits: Reflecting on daily habits reveals insights into lifestyle choices and their impact on diabetes management.
- Positive Discoveries: Discovering positive habits and areas of personal strength fosters a sense of self-empowerment.

2. Health Awareness:

- Increased Consciousness: The past 30 days may have heightened awareness of the connection between choices and overall health.
- Mindful Decision-Making: Acknowledging the power of mindful decision-making in daily life reinforces the importance of health-conscious choices.

3. Support System Appreciation:

- Family and Friends: Reflecting on the support received from family and friends emphasizes the importance of a strong support system.
- Gratitude Expression: Expressing gratitude for the encouragement and understanding of loved ones strengthens the support network.

Setting Intentions for the Future:

1. Building on Success:

- Positive Momentum: Reflecting on achievements sets a positive momentum for the future.
- Building on Success: Identifying successful strategies encourages the continuation of effective habits and practices.

2. Goal Refinement:

- Reassessing Objectives: The end of the past 30 days is an opportune time to reassess goals and refine them based on experiences.
- Clearer Path Forward: A clear vision of refined goals provides a roadmap for the upcoming month.

3. Seeking Continuous Improvement:

- Learning Mindset: Approaching the next phase with a learning mindset ensures a commitment to continuous improvement.
- Adaptive Strategies: Developing adaptive strategies based on past experiences contributes to a proactive and resilient approach.

Recognizing Achievements in the Type 2 Diabetes Journey: A Triumph of Resilience and Determination

Recognizing achievements in the management of Type 2 diabetes is a vital practice that goes beyond acknowledging milestones; it is a celebration of resilience, determination, and the commitment to one's well-being. In this chapter, we delve into the significance of recognizing achievements, the positive impact it has on motivation, and how it contributes to a mindset of empowerment in the face of diabetes management.

Understanding the Significance:

1. Motivational Boost:

- Positive Reinforcement: Recognizing achievements serves as positive reinforcement, providing individuals with the motivation to persist in their diabetes management efforts.
- Mental Well-Being: Regular acknowledgment of successes contributes to a positive mindset, fostering mental well-being.

2. Empowerment and Control:

- Agency in Health: Recognizing achievements reinforces the idea that individuals have agency in their health journey.
- Empowerment: Feeling a sense of control over one's health fosters empowerment and a proactive approach to diabetes management.

3. Building Confidence:

- Self-Belief: Celebrating achievements builds confidence, instilling a belief that individuals can successfully navigate the challenges associated with Type 2 diabetes.
- Self-Efficacy: Recognizing one's ability to make positive changes enhances self-efficacy, contributing to continued efforts.

What Constitutes Achievements in Diabetes Management:

1. Blood Sugar Control:

- Consistent Monitoring: Successfully maintaining consistent blood sugar levels through diligent monitoring is a noteworthy achievement.
- Adaptive Adjustments: Making adaptive adjustments to medication or lifestyle based on blood sugar trends demonstrates proactive management.

2. Lifestyle Modifications:

- Dietary Changes: Any positive adjustments to dietary habits, such as incorporating more whole foods and limiting processed sugars, are significant achievements.
- Physical Activity: Achievements in establishing and sustaining a regular exercise routine contribute to overall well-being.

3. Medication Adherence:

- Consistency: Adhering to prescribed medications consistently is a commendable achievement in maintaining blood sugar control.
- Communication: Openly communicating with healthcare providers about medication experiences and concerns showcases active engagement in one's care.

4. Routine Check-Up Success:

- Positive Feedback: Receiving positive feedback during routine check-ups from healthcare providers indicates successful diabetes management.
- Health Progress: Acknowledging progress in health indicators and test results reflects the effectiveness of efforts.

5. Emotional Resilience:

- Stress Management: Effectively managing stress and incorporating stress-reducing practices is an achievement that positively impacts overall health.
- Mental Health Support: Seeking and utilizing mental health support demonstrates a commitment to emotional well-being.

6. Goal Attainment:

- Setting and Achieving Goals: Whether it's reaching a target HbA1c level or accomplishing small goals, each achievement contributes to the larger picture of success.
- Celebrating Progress: Celebrating progress along the way reinforces the importance of setting and working towards achievable goals.

The Positive Impact on Motivation:

1. Continuous Effort:

- Motivational Momentum: Recognizing achievements creates a positive momentum that fuels continuous effort.
- Feedback Loop: Positive reinforcement from recognizing achievements establishes a feedback loop that propels individuals forward.

2. Intrinsic Motivation:

- Inherent Satisfaction: Intrinsic motivation arises from the inherent satisfaction of recognizing personal achievements.
- Sustainable Drive: This type of motivation is often more sustainable, driving individuals to persist in their diabetes management journey.

3. Overcoming Setbacks:

- Resilience Development: Acknowledging achievements builds resilience, which is crucial for navigating setbacks.
- Learning from Challenges: Viewing setbacks as opportunities for learning and growth contributes to a resilient mindset.

Cultivating a Culture of Recognition:

1. Personal Acknowledgment:

- Self-Celebration: Encouraging individuals to personally acknowledge and celebrate their achievements fosters a culture of self-appreciation.
- Journaling Successes: Maintaining a journal to record achievements allows for reflection and reinforces positive habits.

2. Family and Social Support:

- Shared Celebrations: Involving family and friends in celebrating achievements creates a supportive environment.
- Collective Encouragement: Collective encouragement reinforces the importance of recognizing successes within a social context.

3. Healthcare Provider Involvement:

- Acknowledgment in Consultations: Healthcare providers playing an active role in acknowledging achievements during consultations strengthens the patient-provider relationship.
- Goal-Setting Collaboration: Collaborating with healthcare providers to set achievable goals reinforces a sense of shared responsibility.

Setting Sustainable Long-Term Goals in the Management of Type 2 Diabetes: Building a Foundation for Lasting Well-Being

Setting sustainable long-term goals is a crucial aspect of the journey in managing Type 2 diabetes. Unlike short-term objectives, sustainable goals are enduring and contribute to lasting well-being. This chapter explores the significance of setting such goals, strategies for their establishment, and the positive impact they can have on the overall health and management of Type 2 diabetes.

Understanding the Significance:

1. Continuous Well-Being:

- Holistic Approach: Sustainable long-term goals encompass a holistic approach to well-being, considering physical, mental, and emotional health.
- Enduring Impact: The significance lies in the enduring impact these goals can have on an individual's quality of life.

2. Lifestyle Integration:

- Incorporating Healthy Habits: Sustainable goals involve the incorporation of healthy habits into daily life, making them a natural and integral part of routine.
- Consistent Practice: Long-term goals promote consistent practice, leading to lasting lifestyle changes.

3. Preventive Focus:

- Risk Reduction: Sustainable goals often focus on preventive measures, reducing the risk of complications associated with Type 2 diabetes.
- Long-Term Health: The emphasis is on maintaining long-term health and minimizing the impact of the condition on overall well-being.

Strategies for Establishing Sustainable Goals:

1. Realistic and Achievable:

- Feasibility: Sustainable goals are realistic and achievable, considering individual capabilities, resources, and circumstances.

- Step-by-Step Progress: Breaking down larger goals into smaller, manageable steps ensures a gradual and sustainable approach.

2. Personalized Approach:

- Individual Considerations: Sustainable goals take into account individual preferences, lifestyle, and cultural factors.
- Tailored Strategies: Personalized approaches increase the likelihood of adherence and long-term success.

3. Collaboration with Healthcare Providers:

- Professional Guidance: Involving healthcare providers in goal-setting ensures that objectives align with medical recommendations.
- Regular Assessments: Collaboration allows for regular assessments and adjustments based on health progress.

4. Behavioral Change Techniques:

- Positive Reinforcement: Utilizing positive reinforcement strategies reinforces the adoption of healthy behaviors.
- Cognitive-Behavioral Approaches: Techniques addressing thought patterns and behavior contribute to sustained lifestyle changes.

The Positive Impact on Overall Health:

1. Blood Sugar Control:

- Consistent Management: Sustainable goals contribute to consistent blood sugar control through lifestyle modifications and medication adherence.
- Stabilized Levels: The long-term focus helps in stabilizing blood sugar levels over time.

2. Cardiovascular Health:

- Heart-Healthy Habits: Sustainable goals often include cardiovascular health considerations, promoting heart-healthy habits.
- Risk Reduction: Long-term goals can contribute to reducing the risk of cardiovascular complications associated with Type 2 diabetes.

3. Emotional Well-Being:

- Stress Management: Goals addressing stress reduction and emotional well-being contribute to a more resilient mindset.
- Mental Health Support: Sustainable goals encompass strategies for mental health support, recognizing the interconnectedness of physical and emotional well-being.

4. Weight Management:

- Healthy Weight Maintenance: Long-term goals often involve the maintenance of a healthy weight, reducing the risk of obesity-related complications.
- Nutritious Dietary Practices: Sustainable goals focus on adopting and sustaining nutritious dietary practices for overall health.

5. Physical Activity:

- Regular Exercise: Sustainable goals encourage the incorporation of regular physical activity into daily life.
- Adaptability: Flexibility in exercise routines ensures continued engagement, considering individual preferences and abilities.

Cultivating a Long-Term Mindset:

1. Mindful Decision-Making:

- Conscious Choices: Sustainable goals foster a mindset of mindful decision-making, where choices align with long-term health objectives.
- Reflective Practices: Regular reflection on decisions and their impact supports the cultivation of a long-term mindset.

2. Adaptive Strategies:

- Flexibility: Sustainable goals allow for flexibility, recognizing that life circumstances may change over time.
- Adaptive Approaches: Individuals can adjust strategies based on evolving needs and experiences.

3. Lifelong Learning:

- Ongoing Education: Embracing a mindset of lifelong learning ensures individuals stay informed about the latest advancements in diabetes care.
- Informed Decision-Making: Knowledge empowers informed decision-making for sustained health.

Conclusion

In the pages of "Dealing with Type 2 Diabetes," we have embarked on a comprehensive journey through the intricacies of managing and thriving with Type 2 diabetes. This guide, crafted with care and expertise, serves as a beacon of knowledge, empowerment, and practical strategies for individuals navigating the complex landscape of this chronic condition.

A Holistic Approach to Well-Being:

Throughout this book, we have emphasized the importance of a holistic approach to well-being. From understanding the fundamentals of Type 2 diabetes to delving into the intricacies of insulin resistance and beta cell dysfunction, we have aimed to equip you with a robust foundation of knowledge. This knowledge empowers you to make informed decisions, fostering a sense of agency and control over your health.

Building Lifestyle Foundations:

Lifestyle plays a pivotal role in managing Type 2 diabetes, and our exploration has extended from the impact of lifestyle on diabetes to the nuances of crafting a 30-day meal plan. By providing guidelines for meal planning, sample grocery lists, and quick, healthy recipes, we've sought to make the process of adopting a balanced diet more accessible and enjoyable.

Empowering Through Exercise:

Recognizing the inseparable link between physical activity and diabetes management, we've delved into the benefits of exercise, offering insights into suitable types of exercises and crafting a manageable exercise routine. Understanding the power of regular physical activity is not just about movement; it's about cultivating a lifestyle that embraces vitality and resilience.

Monitoring, Medications, and Emotional Well-Being:

The chapters on monitoring blood sugar levels, medications, and coping with emotional challenges underscore the multifaceted nature of Type 2 diabetes management. From understanding blood glucose meters to exploring coping mechanisms for stress and anxiety, we've provided tools to navigate the emotional terrain that often accompanies this condition.

Preventing Complications and Celebrating Success:

As we explored the importance of routine check-ups, recognizing warning signs, and preventing long-term complications, we've stressed the significance of proactive health management. The journey doesn't just involve avoiding setbacks; it's about celebrating successes, setting future goals, and cultivating a positive mindset that propels you forward.

Reflecting, Recognizing, and Setting Sustainable Goals:

The chapters on reflecting on the past 30 days, recognizing achievements, and setting sustainable long-term goals underscore the transformative power of self-awareness and foresight. By taking stock of your journey, acknowledging achievements, and setting goals that align with your values, you lay the groundwork for enduring health and well-being.

A Comprehensive Guide for Lifelong Wellness:

In conclusion, "Dealing with Type 2 Diabetes" isn't just a book; it's a comprehensive guide crafted to empower you on your journey towards lifelong wellness. Whether you're newly diagnosed, have been managing diabetes for years, or supporting a loved one on this path, our aim has been to provide you with the knowledge, tools, and inspiration needed to navigate the complexities of Type 2 diabetes with resilience and confidence.

Remember, this is not a journey you undertake alone. Your healthcare team, loved ones, and a community of individuals sharing similar experiences stand beside you. The wisdom within these pages is a testament to the strength within you – the strength to adapt, learn, and thrive.

As you continue on this journey, may you find solace in the knowledge gained, inspiration in your achievements, and the resilience to face challenges with unwavering determination. Here's to your health, your well-being, and a future filled with vitality as you navigate the path to wellness with grace and empowerment.

Encouragement and Motivation: A Vital Companion on Your Journey with "Dealing with Type 2 Diabetes"

Embarking on the journey of managing Type 2 diabetes requires not just knowledge but also a wellspring of encouragement and motivation. As you navigate the pages of "Dealing with Type 2 Diabetes," let these words serve as a guiding light, a source of inspiration, and a reminder that you possess the strength to navigate this path with resilience and optimism.

Empowering Knowledge:

Within the chapters of this book, you've immersed yourself in a wealth of empowering knowledge. Remember, knowledge is your ally. It's the compass guiding you through the intricacies of Type 2 diabetes, helping you understand the nuances, make informed decisions, and take charge of your health.

Resilience in Challenges:

In every chapter, we've acknowledged the challenges inherent in managing Type 2 diabetes. From understanding the complexities of insulin resistance to addressing emotional well-being, challenges are part of the journey. Embrace them as opportunities for growth, learning, and resilience. You have within you the power to adapt and overcome.

Fueling Positivity:

Positivity is not just a mindset; it's a fuel that propels you forward. As you explore the benefits of a balanced diet, engage in physical activity, and reflect on your achievements, let positivity be your constant companion. Celebrate your successes, no matter how small, and let them be stepping stones to greater well-being.

Building Habits for Life:

The lifestyle changes explored in this book are not temporary fixes but lifelong habits. Each nutritious meal, every moment of physical activity, and all the choices aligned with your well-being contribute to a healthier, more fulfilling life. Embrace these habits not as restrictions but as opportunities to thrive.

Your Support System:

You're not alone on this journey. Your support system, whether it's family, friends, or a community of individuals sharing similar experiences, is a valuable asset. Lean on them, celebrate with them, and draw strength from their encouragement. Together, you form a collective force against the challenges of Type 2 diabetes.

Setting Goals for Empowerment:

As you set sustainable long-term goals, envision them as markers of empowerment. These goals are not burdens but beacons guiding you towards enduring health. They are your personal roadmaps, filled with milestones that signify progress, growth, and the continuous journey towards optimal well-being.

A Celebration of You:

Consider this book not just a guide but a celebration of you – your strength, resilience, and commitment to a healthier life. Every page turned, every piece of knowledge gained, and every goal set is a testament to your dedication. Recognize your achievements, no matter how small, and let them be sparks that ignite your motivation.

An Ongoing Journey:

Remember, managing Type 2 diabetes is an ongoing journey, and each day is a new opportunity for growth. Embrace the process, learn from experiences, and cultivate a mindset of adaptability. You have the capacity for continuous improvement, and each step forward is a victory in itself.

The Journey Continues:

As you continue with "Dealing with Type 2 Diabetes," let these words be a companion on your journey – a voice of encouragement, a source of motivation, and a reminder that you possess the resilience to navigate the challenges ahead. You are not defined by Type 2 diabetes; rather, you are defined by your strength, your determination, and your commitment to a life filled with vitality and well-being.

Here's to your journey – may it be filled with empowerment, motivation, and the realization of the extraordinary strength within you.

Resources for Ongoing Support: Building a Robust Network for Your Diabetes Journey

Embarking on the path of managing Type 2 diabetes is a journey that benefits from a strong support network and access to valuable resources. Beyond the pages of this book, here's a guide to additional resources that can serve as pillars of ongoing support for you or your loved ones.

1. Healthcare Providers and Diabetes Educators:

Importance:
Your healthcare team is a cornerstone of your diabetes care. They provide medical expertise, guidance on medication management, and insights into crafting a personalized diabetes management plan.

How to Utilize:

- Schedule regular check-ups to monitor your health and discuss any concerns.
- Engage in open communication about your experiences and challenges.
- Seek guidance on lifestyle modifications and medication adjustments.

2. Diabetes Support Groups:

Importance:
Connecting with others who share similar experiences can provide emotional support, encouragement, and a sense of community. Diabetes support groups foster a shared understanding of the challenges and triumphs of living with Type 2 diabetes.

How to Utilize:

- Attend local support group meetings or join online communities.
- Share your experiences and learn from the experiences of others.
- Participate in discussions about coping strategies, lifestyle changes, and successes.

3. Online Communities and Forums:

Importance:

The internet offers a vast array of diabetes-focused platforms where individuals can share information, seek advice, and find support from a global community. Online forums provide a convenient space for connecting with others on a similar journey.

How to Utilize:

- Join reputable diabetes forums and communities.
- Share your questions, concerns, and successes with the community.
- Stay informed about the latest developments in diabetes care.

4. Educational Websites and Apps:

Importance:
Educational websites and apps offer a wealth of information on diabetes management, lifestyle changes, and healthy living. These resources can complement the knowledge gained from healthcare providers and empower individuals to make informed decisions.

How to Utilize:

- Explore reputable websites such as those of diabetes associations and health organizations.
- Download diabetes management apps that help track blood sugar levels, meals, and physical activity.
- Stay informed about the latest research and recommendations.

5. Nutritional Counseling Services:

Importance:
Nutritional counseling can provide personalized guidance on dietary choices, meal planning, and lifestyle modifications. A registered dietitian or nutritionist specializing in diabetes care can offer tailored advice to support your health goals.

How to Utilize:

- Schedule sessions with a registered dietitian or nutritionist.
- Discuss your dietary preferences, challenges, and goals.
- Receive practical advice on creating a balanced and diabetes-friendly meal plan.

6. Mental Health Professionals:

Importance:

The emotional aspects of living with Type 2 diabetes are significant. Mental health professionals, such as psychologists or counselors, can provide support in managing stress, anxiety, and the emotional impact of chronic illness.

How to Utilize:

- Include mental health check-ins as part of your overall healthcare plan.
- Seek support when facing challenges in coping with the emotional aspects of diabetes.
- Learn and practice stress management techniques.

7. Diabetes Associations and Organizations:

Importance:

National and international diabetes associations and organizations offer a wealth of resources, including educational materials, events, and advocacy initiatives. These entities play a vital role in raising awareness and supporting individuals with diabetes.

How to Utilize:

- Explore the resources provided by organizations like the American Diabetes Association, Diabetes UK, or your country's diabetes association.
- Participate in events, campaigns, and initiatives organized by these entities.
- Stay informed about policy changes and advocacy efforts related to diabetes.

8. Exercise and Physical Activity Programs:

Importance:

Regular physical activity is a key component of diabetes management. Participating in exercise programs or working with a fitness professional can provide tailored guidance to enhance your fitness and overall well-being.

How to Utilize:

- Enroll in exercise classes specifically designed for individuals with diabetes.
- Work with a certified fitness trainer experienced in diabetes care.
- Choose physical activities that align with your preferences and health goals.

9. Diabetes Hotlines and Helplines:

Importance:
Hotlines and helplines offer immediate support and guidance. Whether you have urgent questions or need someone to talk to, these resources can be invaluable.

How to Utilize:

- Save the numbers of diabetes hotlines for quick access.
- Use helplines during moments of uncertainty or when seeking immediate advice.

10. Books, Literature, and Educational Materials:

Importance:
Educational materials, including books, pamphlets, and brochures, can provide in-depth insights into various aspects of diabetes. These resources serve as valuable references for ongoing learning.

How to Utilize:

- Build a library of diabetes-related literature for continuous education.
- Refer to reputable books and materials recommended by healthcare professionals.
- Stay updated on new publications in the field.

Additional Resources:

Thank you for choosing "Dealing with Type 2 Diabetes" as your guide to a healthier and more empowered life. For ongoing support, updates, and exclusive content, we invite you to visit our Author Central page on Amazon. Here, you'll find:

- Author Insights: Gain deeper insights into the book, its creation, and ongoing health-related content directly from Dr. Edna Swindell.
- Community Engagement: Join discussions, share your experiences, and connect with a community of individuals on a similar journey to manage and thrive with Type 2 diabetes.
- Exclusive Content: Access bonus materials, additional recipes, and the latest information on managing diabetes and improving overall well-being.

Your journey to optimal health is important, and our Author Central page is designed to be a hub of resources to support you every step of the way.

Visit our Author Central page on Amazon:

www.ednaswindell.com